Study Guide for

Care Support Workers

Level 2

NVQ/SVQ in Care

Mandatory Group A and Option Group B Units

Stephen O'Kell

First Class Books, Inc.
P.O. Box 1, Portishead
Bristol, BS20 9 BR

Study Guide for
Care Support Workers
Level 2

ISBN: 1-880246-11-2

Copyright © October, 1999
by First Class Books, Inc.

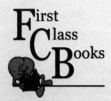

First
Class
Books

P.O. Box 1, Portishead
Bristol BS20 9BR

Phone: (01823) 323 126
Fax: (01823) 321 876

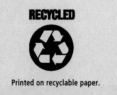

RECYCLED

Printed on recyclable paper.

Introduction

The new level 2 National Vocational Qualification/Scottish Vocational Qualification (NVQ/SVQ) in Care Award provides a set of performance standards for Care Support Workers from all occupational groups. The care standards specify the quality of performance in the workplace for those people who deliver hands-on care. Achieving the standards develops competence for assisting care professionals in institutional and community settings.

The award consists of mandatory and optional units. Mandatory units are common to all the NVQ/SVQ in Care awards undertaken at level 2 and, therefore, must be completed by all candidates. Optional units are those which are most relevant to an individual's work role that a candidate can choose to complete an NVQ/SVQ award.

To achieve the full award (nine units), a candidate must complete all four Mandatory Group A units plus five optional units. At least three of the optional units must be chosen from Option Group B. If required, the remainder can be chosen from Option Group C (maximum 2 units). This workbook provides the underpinning knowledge relating to the four Mandatory Group A units and the ten Option Group B units of the level 2 NVQ/SVQ in Care award.

Contents

 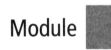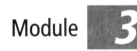

Fostering Equality and Diversity

Promote equal opportunities and rights for all.

Need-to-know words:

- abuse
- adopted role
- advocate
- ascribed role
- assault
- assertive
- at risk
- battery
- challenging behaviour
- confidentiality
- defamation
- depersonalisation
- discrimination
- diversity
- empathy
- equality
- false documentation
- halo effect
- institutionalisation
- label
- libel
- negligence
- noncompliance
- paranoia
- prejudice
- prognosis
- rights
- significant other
- slander
- stereotype
- stigma

Objectives:

- Outline how to foster the rights of others.
- Highlight the potential for conflict between individual roles and responsibilities.
- Respect the personal beliefs and life choices of others.
- Recognise the various forms of discrimination and their effect on the provision of care.
- Describe how equality can be promoted in care environments.
- Describe how to maintain confidentiality.
- Identify causes of challenging behaviour.
- Describe the different types of abuse and signs and symptoms of abuse.
- Utilise a model for analysing challenging behaviour.
- Outline how to care for people "at risk."

Module 1 Introduction

Module 1 relates directly to two units of the level 2 NVQ/SVQ Award in Care:

Unit O1: **Promote people's equality, diversity, and rights** is a mandatory group A unit that consists of three elements of competence:

- O1.1 Foster people's rights and responsibilities.
- O1.2 Foster equality and diversity of people.
- O1.3 Maintain the confidentiality of information.

Unit Z1: **Contribute to the protection of individuals from abuse** is also a mandatory group A unit which consists of three elements of competence:

- Z1.1 Contribute to minimising the level of abuse in environments.
- Z1.2 Minimise the effects of abusive behaviour.
- Z1.3 Contribute to monitoring individuals who are at risk from abuse.

Part 1: Promoting Rights and Responsibilities (O1.1)

Promote and support individual rights and choices.

People have many ethical and legal rights within the United Kingdom. The **Universal Declaration of Human Rights** (United Nations, 1948) has had considerable impact throughout the world. The declaration includes the following rights:

- Recognition as a person before the law
- Education and employment
- Self-determination
- Life
- Not being subjected to medical experimentation without consent
- Social security
- Adequate standard of living including food, clothing, and housing

The **Declaration of Rights of Mentally Retarded Persons** (United Nations, 1971) recognised that people who have learning disabilities might not be adequately covered by the previous declaration. It states that people who have learning disabilities should have the same rights as other people, insofar as this is feasible, and guardians (advocates) should be appointed if they cannot make their own decisions.

The **Mental Health Act** (United Nations, 1983) addresses the following legal rights:

- Voting
- Entering hire purchase contracts
- Entering into marriage
- Having property and assets protected
- Having protection against cruelty and exploitation
- Writing to certain members of society

The **law of the land** gives citizens further rights:

- To vote
- To demonstrate
- To legal representation
- To protection from theft and physical harm

Exercise 1.1 🖉

Care in the Community guidelines were established by the Department of Health (1990) for local authorities to be responsible for planning the provision of community care services in their localities.

Local authorities work in conjunction with the following:

- District health authorities
- Primary care groups
- Local housing authorities
- Voluntary organisations
- Private sector care organisations

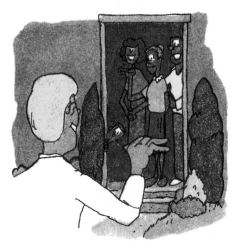

Community services have been established so that, where possible, people who need care in the community have a right to available services:

- A full assessment of needs and the delivery of a negotiated package of services to meet those needs
- Domiciliary, day, and respite services to enable people to live in their own homes, where feasible and sensible
- Practical support for families who provide care for relatives at home
- Residential care services for individuals who cannot cope on their own

The **Patient's Charter** clearly sets out people's rights to care and standards of service that should be provided by the NHS, GP, hospital, community, ambulance, dental, optical, and pharmaceutical services. A health authority's performance in relation to the Patient's Charter standards is important because the Department of Health compares its performance to those of other health authorities and publicly reports on its findings in the form of performance league tables each year.

The Patient's Charter will eventually be replaced by a new set of national standards and guidelines which will be backed by a National Institute for Clinical Excellence and a Commission for Health Improvement. The commission will have the power to intervene when health care is not available to acceptable standards (Department of Health, 1997).

Exercise 1.2

Promote and support the rights of each person in your care. Encourage them to express their needs and wishes. When individuals make choices, this encourages their independence.

- Stick to your promises, and inform people if you are going to be late.
- Be specific when providing options to clients. Let them know if the options are restricted. Explain why, and make a record of the transaction.
- If, for any reason, someone is unable to make choices, take the person's interests into account before making a choice for the person. Do this by consulting others (e.g., advocate, friend, relative, significant other, interpreter) before you make the decision.
- Give a clear explanation when a person's request cannot be granted or must be restricted.
- Do not allow yourself or others to be manipulated.
- If you have concerns about offering choices, seek advice.

Some client groups are much more likely to be deprived of their rights to available services because of the effects of prejudice and because they may not actively seek services (e.g., gypsies, tramps, New-Age travellers, some ethnic minorities). The emphasis for these groups must be on informing them of available services and ensuring accessibility to those services.

Responsibilities

A person's responsibilities are usually dependent on that individual's roles in life and in society as a whole. The following roles provide responsibilities for people which may be difficult for them to carry out when they are ill, disabled, or require care:

- Family roles (e.g., father, sister, uncle, grandparent)

- Work roles (e.g., heavy lifting, typing)

- Legal roles (e.g., juror, guardian, tax payer)

- Societal roles (e.g., good neighbour, breadwinner)

- Religious roles (e.g., attending mass, fasting during Ramadan)

- Social roles (e.g., footballer, choirmaster, scout)

An inability to carry out any of the above ascribed or adopted roles can be very stressful for that person and any others who are dependent on that role being carried out.

Exercise 1.3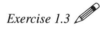

Sometimes there can be conflicts in people's roles and responsibilities. Following are examples:

- Between the different roles in a person's life (e.g., long hours at work may make it difficult to spend much time with the family)

- Between one's own rights and responsibilities (e.g., caring for a sick relative may prevent a person from continuing his or her education or gaining employment)

- Between the rights and responsibilities of different people (e.g., a nurse's responsibility to give medication and a patient's right to refuse it)

- Between the rights and responsibilities of individuals and organisations (e.g., the right for personal information to be kept confidential against an organisation's responsibility to ensure access to that information by a number of professionals)

Exercise 1.4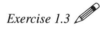

Individual Rights

It is essential that you promote the rights of all the people in your care. They must come first—usually before you and your employing organisation. Make sure that you know your organisations's policies relating to people's rights, including your responsibilities and the boundaries of action that you can take.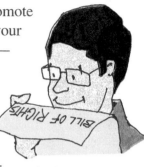

You need to be aware of your own values and beliefs so that you can ensure that they do not conflict with your expected work roles. If you have difficulties in this area (e.g., your work uniform does not conform to the requirements of your religion to cover parts of your body), consult your manager.

The promotion of individual rights can be achieved in a number of ways:

- Reminding individuals of their rights (e.g., to welfare benefits)

- Identifying and assessing individuals who are incapacitated to make sure that they are receiving their rights, or advocating on their behalf when necessary (e.g., insisting that an individual does not have too many visitors when adequate rest is essential to the person's care)

- Ensuring that individuals who cannot speak up for themselves have interpreters or advocates to represent them and ensure that their rights are met

- Ensuring that information relating to rights and resources or support is made available to people (e.g., providing information leaflets, showing people how to use the complaints system, referring people to colleagues or departments where relevant information is available, directing individuals to the Citizens Advice Bureau)

- Informing your manager when a person's rights are being infringed, especially if local policies are not being followed or when there may be legal implications
- Gently challenging people when their choices of action infringe on the rights of others (e.g., requesting an angry relative, who is complaining about the quality of care, to accompany you to the office so that he or she does not frighten or disturb others)

Exercise 1.5 ✏

Part 2: Promoting Equality and Diversity (01.2)

Treat everyone with respect and dignity.

When people meet others for the first time, they tend to make assumptions about them. The assumptions will be based on whether the people are similar to, or different from, them. Depending on their own values, attitudes, and beliefs (value position), they may view the differences positively or negatively. A value position acts like a filter in the perception of facts about others.

Personal Beliefs and Identity

To respect the personal beliefs and identity of others, you need to be aware of your own value position. You will also need to develop the ability to shift your (value) position in order to see things from the points of view of others—putting yourself in their shoes. This will enable you to appreciate the different perspectives (values, attitudes, and beliefs) of others so that you can develop empathy when caring for these people.

You will be expected to recognise and support individual beliefs and preferences. Actively encourage people in your care to express their beliefs, wishes, and views, as long as they do not interfere with the rights of others. Personal beliefs and preferences are important. Therefore, acknowledge individuals' beliefs about self, race, religion, politics, culture, ethics, and sexuality by responding in a manner that is supportive.

Also, be aware of your own beliefs if they are likely to cause conflict in the provision of care (e.g., if you are a strict Catholic, you will not want to be involved in abortions). Inform your supervisor if your care role conflicts with your religious or other beliefs.

Beliefs and preferences affect the foods people eat, the clothing they wear, how they worship, and other aspects of daily living. You can support an individual's beliefs in a variety of ways:

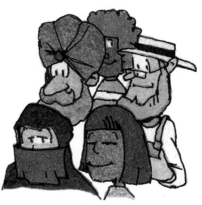

- Be sensitive to each person's needs.
- Support the right to practice individual beliefs.
- Make sure your speech and actions do not offend others.
- Address individuals by their preferred names and titles.
- Take into consideration beliefs and lifestyles when planning care.
- Be respectful of each person's customs and possessions.
- Show interest in each person's beliefs.
- Be willing to listen when a person wants to talk.
- Never question or make fun of another person's beliefs.

9

- Never try to force your beliefs on another person.
- Never ask non-Christians for their "Christian names." (Ask for their first names.)

Exercise 1.6 ✎

Religious Customs

Be familiar with religious customs (e.g., Sikh men must leave their hair unshorn and wear a turban). The more you know, the less likely you 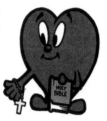 are to offend someone. People may have religious items in their possession (such as rosaries or prayer books). If you must move these items, handle them with respect.

Holidays: Be aware of days that are celebrated with special rituals (e.g., Passover for Jews). People may need extra help dressing for holidays or they may need privacy for certain rituals (e.g., confession or prayer).

Foods: Some religions forbid certain foods. Know what is not allowed, and offer other choices. (For example, most Moslems and Hindus do not eat pork or beef; they only eat meat that has been killed a special way). Be aware of special times that people may eat only certain foods (e.g., Ramadan for Moslems) or fast (go without food) .

Clothing: Some religions have certain articles of clothing that must be worn or treated with respect (e.g., devout Moslem women may leave only their eyes uncovered in public).

Medical treatments: Be aware of any medical treatments that are not allowed because of religious beliefs (e.g., blood transfusions for Jehovah's Witness followers).

Clergy: If an individual wants to see a member of clergy, make sure all relevant people are informed. Provide privacy whenever a member of the clergy visits.

Death: Different religions have different rules governing what to do with a body after death (e.g., followers of Islam should not be touched by non-Moslems after death; if they have to be touched, wear gloves).

Exercise 1.7 ✎

Discrimination

Always provide quality care, regardless of a person's background, beliefs, race, ethnicity, gender, sexuality, age, mental or physical ability. Your personal beliefs and preferences should not affect the quality of service you provide. Your personal beliefs can affect your behaviour in a variety of direct and indirect ways.

Be aware of legislation and local organisational policies that prohibit discriminatory practice (unfair treatment). The Disability Discrimination Act (1995) makes it unlawful to discriminate unjustifiably against disabled people.

The ways in which you communicate with people should reflect your care role and the power invested in that role. Therefore, if you have any feelings of hostility toward population groups, be careful not to express those feelings at work. If necessary, seek advice on how to deal with your feelings.

There are different types of discrimination. *Overt discrimination* operates when a person is openly discriminating (e.g., advertising that your club is only open to white-skinned people). *Covert discrimination* is much more difficult to prove. An example is when all the managers of an organisation who have risen through the ranks are males, when the majority of employees are females.

Appropriate discrimination can take the form of refusing to employ convicted child abusers to work in a children's home, or not allowing children with epilepsy to play on the high climbing frame. *Inappropriate* (but not illegal) *discrimination* can take the form of employing only people under the age of 55 years into senior management posts. Another example is accepting unnecessarily rude and aggressive behaviour from a disabled person, just because he or she is disabled.

Exercise 1.8

To promote equality, it is important to recognise and accept other people's beliefs and lifestyles (even when they clash with your own). Every individual has the right to equality and an acceptable quality of life, regardless of the person's past history and beliefs.

Stereotyping and Prejudice

Many groups of people have stereotypes attached to them on the basis that people from the same groups have similar characteristics or traits (e.g., Scots are mean, redheads are fiery, accountants are boring). Therefore, people sometimes attribute a variety of qualities or labels to an individual that are radically wrong.

Some stereotypes have positive values attached to them, and some have negative values attached, referred to as a *stigma*. A person with a stigma is often a target for discrimination. In the care sector, there are several client groups that carry a stigma (e.g., people who are elderly, disabled, mentally ill, or who have learning disabilities).

This stigma leads to the *halo effect* where there is a strong tendency for these people to conform to others' negative expectations of them. People's negative expectations tend to affect the quality of their interactions with these stigmatised individuals, further reducing chances for improved relationships.

Equal Opportunities

The Equal Opportunities Commission (1986) outlined 10 aspects that should be written into organisational policies if they are to become equal opportunity employers. The policies should include the following:

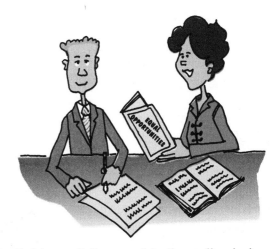

- Definitions of direct and indirect discrimination, victimisation, and sexual harassment
- A statement of the organisation's commitment to equal opportunities
- The name of the officer(s) responsible for ensuring the policy is carried out
- Details for how the policy is to be carried out
- An obligation upon employees to respect and act in accordance with the policy
- Procedures for dealing with complaints of discrimination
- Examples of unlawful practices
- Details of monitoring and reviewing procedures
- A commitment to remove barriers to equal opportunity
- Provision of equal opportunities training

Protect yourself and others from discrimination by taking appropriate action. Provide feedback to anyone who has been discriminatory; explain the effects and consequences of his or her actions. Offer support and guidance to people who have been discriminated against and to those at risk of discrimination. Make a formal complaint about any discrimination you encounter, or support others in doing so.

Exercise 1.9

Part 3: Maintaining Confidentiality (01.3)

Ensure right of access before disclosing personal details about clients.

In the course of your work, you will need to handle health and care records. The confidential nature of these records cannot be overstressed. Information about the people in your care is very private.

Individuals have a right to expect that information given in confidence will be used only for the purpose for which it was given and that it will not be released to others without their consent.

Confidential information includes all medical information—diagnosis, prognosis, and treatment—and everything related to personal, social, and financial data. The person-in-charge of your part of the organisation has the responsibility for maintaining the security of all health, care, and service provision records.

You have both a legal and moral responsibility to maintain confidentiality about personal information. Information is disclosed only to those who have the right and the need to know, according to statutory or agency policies. Never disclose information unless you have proof of the enquirer's identity and right of access. Unauthorized disclosure or misuse of information contained in health and care records is a serious breach of discipline and could lead to your dismissal.

Make sure that you know your organisation's policies that pertain to your role relating to confidentiality, access, and transmission of information. This includes knowing the records that can be accessed by people receiving care and those to which they should not have access. For example, it is appropriate that a patient/client should have access to his or her own plan of care, but not to budget sheets or the accident book for a particular establishment.

Exercise 1.10 🖉

The United Kingdom Central Council for Nursing, Midwifery, and Health Visiting (1987) provides general guidelines on confidentiality, emphasizing accountability for confidential information obtained in the course of practice.

The **Data Protection Act** (Home Office, 1998) establishes the principles for managing electronically-held information and structured paper-based, client records. These principles specify that personal data must meet the following criteria:

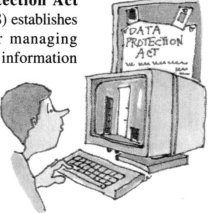

- Processed fairly and lawfully with special care being taken with sensitive, personal data
- Obtained only for lawful purposes, as specified in the Act
- Be adequate, relevant, and not excessive for the specified purposes
- Be accurate and, where necessary, kept up-to-date
- Kept no longer than necessary for the specified purposes
- Ensure an individual's rights (e.g., making a person's records available to him or her upon request)
- Properly protected against loss or disclosure
- Not be transferred to countries outside the European Economic Community

The Act also clearly specifies a number of offences which include unlawfully obtaining or selling personal data, unlawfully accessing data via a third party, and unlawfully disclosing information to others.

The **Access to Health Records Act** (NHSME, 1990) provides anyone over 16 years of age with the right to see his or her health records unless there are compelling reasons to deny access. Health records are defined as any record concerning the physical or mental health of an individual who can be identified from the information recorded (e.g., details of investigations, diagnosis, treatment, or examinations). The Act allows for an individual to apply to access his or her own health records. This is achieved by writing to the holder of the record (e.g., doctor or health authority). The application must be fully processed within 40 days, and a fee plus the cost of postage and copying may be charged (unless the applicant simply reads the records on the spot).

Exercise 1.11 🖉

Following is the **Code of Practice**:

- Records should be handled only by staff authorised to handle them as part of their duties.

- The contents of health and care records should never, under any circumstances, be communicated to persons who are not authorised to have them.

- The contents of records should be discussed only with persons who need to know in order to carry out their care roles.

- If you find someone who is unknown to you who is handling or reading health or care records, challenge the person for proof of identity and authority to handle the records.

- Record stores should be kept locked when not in use, with the key being held by an authorised person.

- Electronic access codes to databases should be kept secret by the carers who have been given the authority to use the codes.

Breaching Confidentiality

There may be times when you are told information that needs to be passed on to someone else for action (e.g., when someone is at risk). You will need to check your organisation's policies relating to this issue.

When you must pass on information that has been given to you in confidence, carefully explain to the person who told you that you may have to share the information with others (e.g., when you find out that a person is a substance abuser or is contemplating suicide). Explain the reasons why the information should be shared with others and who, precisely, will have access to the information.

In addition, conflict can arise between confidentiality and the legal need to share information with other parties (e.g., the police). The Data Protection Act allows personal data to be disclosed to certain parties when it is essential for the purposes of preventing or detecting a crime or for the apprehension or prosecution of offenders.

Confidentiality can be inadvertently breached when members of staff are not careful with confidential information. It may occur when talking about clients in corridors, on public transport, etc., where other people can hear. Case notes may be left lying around where unauthorised people can simply pick them up and read them, or personal information may be left unattended on computer screens for unauthorised people to read.

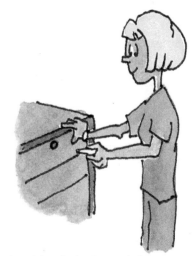

If you see or hear a breach of confidentiality, take action immediately. Lock case notes away. Blank out computer screens, or turn the screens so that unauthorised people cannot see them. Courteously point out to the people concerned that they are breaching confidentiality, that they should refrain from doing so, and that they are putting their jobs at risk if they are caught or reported. If confidentiality is being blatantly breached, despite warnings, report the people concerned to an appropriate manager.

Part 4: Protecting Individuals from Abuse (Z1)

Help to minimise the level of abuse.

It is important to understand that there is always a reason for a person's behaviour. People receiving care are often adjusting to changes in their lifestyles that affect them physically, emotionally, and socially.

People receiving care nowadays are much more knowledgable about care services and their rights. Not everyone's expectations can be met, which has led to a general increase in abuse and aggression toward care workers.

Today's faster pace of life and social problems result in more people suffering from the effects of stress, and individuals cope with their frustrations in different ways. Some people take out their anger on everyone; others may be quiet and withdrawn. Some people blame all of their problems on others; others blame themselves. Some deny there is a problem; others try to find a reason for everything.

Never express anger or irritation toward the people in your care. Your attitude affects their behaviour and well-being. Understanding and accepting your own feelings is important. Whenever you feel frustrated, try to understand why you feel that way. If you are unable to cope with your feelings, seek advice.

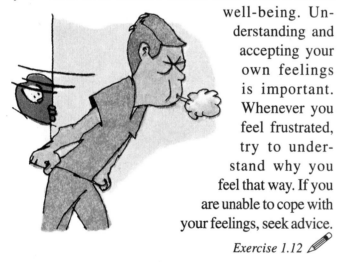

Exercise 1.12 🖉

To manage abusive behaviour, the emphasis must be on prevention and de-escalation of the situation before aggression occurs. Abuse aimed at care staff is often caused by an action, or a failure to carry out an action, by a member of the care staff.

In addition, avoid personal behaviour which can provoke or escalate abuse.

- Avoid using a tone of voice that is nagging, demanding, or showing boredom.
- Do not break off conversations without apologising, and always try to return to a conversation after an interruption.
- Do not overreact by using abusive language or issuing threats.
- Avoid getting into arguments.
- Do not ignore questions or the people posing them.
- Try to remain calm.
- Although abuse is personal in nature, do not take it personally.
- Accept apologies gracefully.
- Do not use phrases such as "calm down" or "don't be silly" as these talk down to the person and belittle the problem.
- Avoid laughing, chatting, reading magazines, etc., in front of people who are waiting.
- Use appropriate non-verbal communication. Do not shrug your shoulders, raise your eyebrows, point, commence clock watching, stand with your hands on your hips or arms folded across your chest, etc.
- Do not point at, or push, an abuser.
- Maintain a normal distance between yourself and the abuser.
- Try to get the abuser to sit down and talk.

Exercise 1.13 🖉

Challenging Behaviour

Sometimes people are uncooperative, demanding, threatening, rude, or stubborn. Try to find the underlying cause of the behaviour. Some common concerns that affect people's behaviour include the following:

- Anxiety, fear
- Change in lifestyle
- Health problems
- Depression
- Loneliness
- Physical and mental changes
- Lack of understanding
- Family problems
- Religious concerns
- Pain
- Grief
- Unmet needs
- Financial concerns
- Loss of independence
- Longing for the "old days"
- Unmet expectations
- Lack of self-esteem
- Lack of sleep or rest

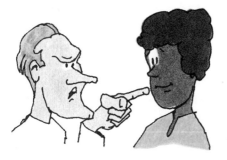

Occasionally, people become angry or upset about the situation of their loved one. Even though it can be difficult for you, try to be understanding and supportive of these people.

Abuse in the form of discrimination can occur if people are labeled as "difficult," "awkward," or a "problem." Sometimes carers try to avoid these people, and this can make them more abusive.

Exercise 1.14

Timing and mood are important variables which can make people react differently to the same stimulus at different times. For example, a person might be happy to listen to a long-winded joke most of the time, but it might make the person quite angry if you try telling the joke when he or she is rushing to make an appointment or when feeling ill.

Be aware of other factors that can cause challenging behaviour:

- The influence of alcohol or drugs (prescribed or illegal)
- Mental illness, especially when there are feelings of paranoia
- The environment (e.g., noisy, dirty, crowded, hot)
- The affect of having to wait and/or queue for long lengths of time
- Your dress and professional manner, (representing unacceptable "authority")
- Your irritating behaviour (e.g., showing boredom, interrupting others' conversations)

Exercise 1.15

Challenging behaviour can often be reduced by offering advice and support, as appropriate, to help people understand why their inappropriate behaviour may be seen as abusive. Use your interpersonal skills to deflect people's energies into useful activity rather than escalating conflict.

Abuse

Abuse refers to any situation where a person's human or legal rights are refused, restricted, or curtailed. People who are close to a person being abused often do not know and will not allow themselves to believe that it is happening. They may become very upset about the suspicions of care staff.

Abuse can take many forms and be short-term or long-term. It can be difficult to identify. For example, when does corporal punishment of a child become physical abuse, and when does a husband's bad temper become psychological abuse?

Abuse can be categorised according to the abuser—*self-abuse* (e.g., taking illegal drugs, purposeful self-injury) and *other abuse* (e.g., child abuse, granny bashing).

Abuse can also be categorised according to the nature of the abuse that has taken place:

- **Physical abuse** (e.g., physical injuries from an attack or injuries caused by lack of an awareness of danger)
- **Sexual abuse** (e.g., rape, indecent assault, allowing a child to watch blue movies)
- **Psychological abuse** (e.g., creating anxiety over a period of time by the use of threats, not allowing a person to meet other people, institutionalisation)

Exercise 1.16 ✐

Signs and Symptoms of Abuse

It is possible for the signs and symptoms of abuse to occur when there has been no abuse. Suspicion usually occurs when several of the signs and symptoms are noticed at once and over time. This may be linked to explanations that are inconsistent with the injury or behaviour. Many of the short-term effects of abuse are well-documented. However, the long-term effects can be more traumatic, especially if the victim exhibits behaviour that makes other people reject him or her.

Physical signs and symptoms:

- Multiple bruises/bruises of different ages
- Bruises on the face, especially around the mouth and ears
- Splits on the inside of lips
- Fingertip bruising (resulting from having been forcibly gripped)
- Bite marks (usually an oval bruise with a gap at each side)
- Odd-shaped bruises that outline the shape of the weapon used
- Scratch marks and bruises in difficult-to-injure places (e. g., inner thigh, inner or upper arm)
- Burns and scalds (cigarette burns cause a round mark or scar one to one and one-half centimetres across)

- Injuries and infections of the genitals
- General signs of neglect (including poor standards of hygiene and general nutrition)
- Munchausen syndrome by proxy (where the parent deliberately fabricates a child's symptoms in order to obtain surgery for the child)

Psychological signs and symptoms:

- Withdrawal and depression (avoiding eye contact, passivity, no spontaneous smiles)

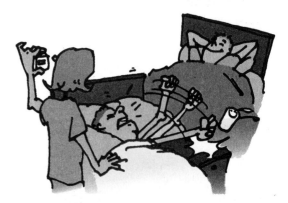

- Inappropriate/unacceptable behaviour (avoidance or attention-seeking behaviour, tantrums, aggression)
- Anxiety (jumpy, tense, "frightened eyes")
- Impaired capacity to enjoy life
- Symptoms of psychiatric illness

Whether a person is abused in an isolated incident or over a prolonged period of time by one or many people, it is impossible to forecast what the long-term effects will be.

Exercise 1.17 ✐

Managing Abuse

Whenever serious abuse is suspected, a person can be admitted to hospital or taken to a "place of safety" for observation so that a more comprehensive assessment can be carried out. The most important aspects of caring for people who have been abused are listed on the following page.

- Recognising the signs and symptoms of abuse
- Making accurate records of what you observe or what is reported by the client
- Informing an appropriate person of any concerns that you may have
- Ensuring that you know the plan of care for the abused person (this may include monitoring the person's whereabouts, placing restrictions on the person's movements, or restricting access to the person by potential visitors)
- Offering advice to the person on how to avoid or minimise the level of abuse

Exercise 1.18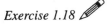

Minimising Challenging Behaviour

Try to minimise the negative effects of disruptive and abusive behaviour. To do this, it is essential that you understand the cause of challenging behaviour before attempting to do anything to prevent or manage it (Poyner & Warne, 1988). The model below allows for an analysis to be made of all incidents of challenging behaviour. It consists of a carer interacting with a care recipient in a care environment to produce an outcome (challenging behaviour).

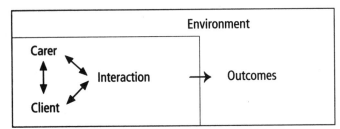

Model for Understanding Challenging Behaviour

The Carer

The characteristics of the carer can have a significant effect on the outcomes of care provision.

Appearance and first impressions are important in any job involving encounters with the public.

For example, a uniform can prevent some people from being abusive and may stimulate others to be abusive.

Tolerance to stress may be important for your success in dealing with difficult interactions (e.g., your ability to control a group of boisterous children can be impaired if you are stressed by illness or work overload).

Experienced staff have usually experienced similar situations, and the expectation is that they are more likely to handle challenging behaviour more effectively.

Gender inevitably has an influence on challenging behaviour. For example, a woman might find it easier than a man to calm down an angry man, although women tend to feel more vulnerable to attack in certain situations.

Personality and temperament of the carer affect behaviour. Some carers appear to be naturally better at handling difficult situations, usually because they have good interpersonal skills.

Attitude toward people who need care and their families, and attitude to the job role tend to have an effect on how a carer behaves toward the people in his or her care.

Expectations that carers have about their jobs influence their ability to handle difficult situations. For example, a carer who always expects people to conform to the plan of care is likely to cause anger and resentment in people who do not agree with the planned care.

Exercise 1.19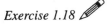

The behaviour of the carer can also have a significant impact on the level of abuse experienced.

Treat people with respect and dignity. Do not "talk down" to people. Appear confident and concerned; avoid pat responses (e.g., "Everything will be alright"). Evaluate your own performance during interactions with people who are being abusive.

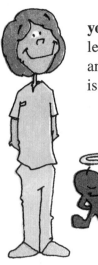

Maintain personal control of your feelings. Remain calm, regardless of the situation. Showing your anger or displeasure at another person is likely to escalate the conflict.

Be honest with people. Although it is important to control your anger, it is sometimes necessary to reveal your personal feelings. Communicate openly and effectively to promote acceptance and trust.

Provide face-saving alternatives. Be willing to bargain and compromise by providing care alternatives from which a person can choose. This promotes a willingness to accept the care being provided. For example, a person complaining about the timing of meals could be offered alternative eating arrangements.

Set limits to behaviour. Communicate clear messages about what is expected. Be consistently firm, and be assertive where necessary, (e.g., asking a person to stop smoking in a room that is clearly marked with "no smoking" signs).

Promote expression of feelings. Allow and acknowledge feelings of anger or fear, and encourage the safe expression of those feelings. When appropriate, allowing a person the chance to "let off steam" may prevent the problem from escalating to violence.

Monitor people's behaviour. The care worker continually assesses the environment so that he or she can choose the right moment and right manner to intervene. Monitoring involves recognising patterns of behaviour and getting to know the people who are receiving care. Especially important is being sensitive to non-verbal behaviours exhibited by both yourself and others.

Provide time to calm down. Give a person time to calm down or to talk through the problem. Getting the person to describe the problem helps to refocus thinking on the problem rather than on acting out the anger, and it often provides the essential "cooling down period."

Exercise 1.20

The Client

The characteristics of the client can also have a significant effect on the outcomes of care provision.

Personality and temperament of the care recipient affect behaviour. Some environments have to be set up specifically for care recipients who are likely to exhibit challenging behaviour (e.g., acute psychiatric units, substance abuse units, welfare benefit offices).

Temporary conditions affect care, such as care recipients who are under the influence of drugs or alcohol, suffering from an illness, or distressed.

Negative or uncertain expectations of the interaction to come can impact the situation. For example, a daughter expects that her father cannot be provided with care to meet his needs, and she is deeply concerned that he cannot remain in his own home.

Immaturity can be a problem; children cannot be expected to control their emotions and behaviour.

Exercise 1.21

The Environment

Environment is the total context in which the care service is delivered. Each environment has factors which have an effect on incidents of challenging behaviour. Consider the following factors:

- **Working alone**: Home visits by health and social services staff are more difficult because the care worker is a guest in people's homes, and there is no back-up if things go wrong.

- **Job location**: Locally-based care services are usually better able to respond sympathetically to difficult situations because they are aware of local issues. A care worker who provides services in a very rough area of town is more likely to encounter aggressive behaviour.

- **Cash or drugs being carried**: Care workers are potential targets for robbers.
- **Waiting and queuing**: These are two of the many hassles with which the public has to cope.
- **Time**: People are more likely to be drunk at certain times, and children are more likely to be on the streets at certain times of the day/week.
- **Territory**: People feel more comfortable in their own territory. This can affect the chances of challenging behaviour occurring.
- **Room design**: This includes room temperature, available space, seating arrangements, decorations, and furniture, etc. High room temperatures are much more likely to make people drowsy, irritable, and aggressive.

Exercise 1.22

The Interaction

If a person believes that he or she is being treated in an unfair or unreasonable way, it is not unusual for challenging behaviour to occur. Challenging behaviour can vary between difficult-to-handle behaviours (e.g., non-compliance, verbal abuse, spitting) to physical assault and violence.

If you are monitoring and recording a person's behaviour, try not to make it obvious, or you may get inaccurate results and/or make matters worse. Make accurate and complete records of all incidents of challenging behaviour.

Assertiveness refers to your ability to express your views in a clear, confident, and direct manner without denying the rights of others. Assertive behaviour is always preferable to passive or aggressive behaviour. Your clear, confident, and direct manner means that you can resolve problems without resorting to threats or manipulation. It also allows you to handle criticisms and uncertainty calmly. Furthermore, assertion can help you to refuse requests without feeling guilty or to ask for help when it is needed without feeling inadequate.

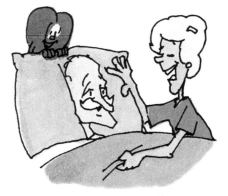

The following assertion techniques can be used as a means of handling abusive and aggressive behaviour (Wondrak, 1989):

- **Self-disclosure**: Admitting that you are afraid
- **Partial agreement**: Agreeing with part of a person's criticism (e.g., "Yes, l could have handled the situation a little better, but l am happy with the way things have turned out.")
- **Gentle confrontation**: Confronting a person in an attempt to uncover the reason for the abusive behaviour (e.g., "I am sorry. I did not mean to upset you by opening all the upstairs windows. What is the problem?")
- **Side stepping**: Agreeing fully with a person's criticism (e.g., "Yes, it was silly to close all the windows when it is so hot.")
- **Being specific**: Keeping what you have to say as specific as possible and avoiding unnecessary waffle (e.g., "John, I notice you keep kicking Jane under the table.")

Exercise 1.23

Understand your employer's policies regarding the management of aggression and violence. It is the employer's duty under the Health and Safety at Work Act (1974) to ensure that the work environment is as safe as possible for employees. Examples include visible security systems for buildings where appropriate, adequate staffing, and appropriate training to handle aggression and violence (Health and Safety Commission, 1987).

Exercise 1.24

Monitoring "At-Risk" Individuals

It is your duty to report all complaints and any suspected abuse. In addition, it is your legal responsibility to respect people's rights and to protect them from harm (e.g., assault, battery, defamation, false documentation, negligence). Legal action may result from abuse or failure to report suspected abuse.

The most common type of abuse is child abuse. Each area of the country has local professional guidelines for referring children who are suspected of being abused. Your point of referral will probably be to discuss your concerns with your manager, who will decide whether to refer the matter to a statutory agency.

Child abuse may not be the only type of abuse that you come across. If any person in your care complains about having been abused or if you suspect abuse, report your evidence immediately to the person-in-charge. Make a detailed written record in your own handwriting while details are still fresh in your memory. The handwritten record should be retained (even if the report is eventually typed) as it can be used as evidence in court.

If a person in your care needs protection from abuse, be sure that you know the care plan and any rules or regulations that pertain to the situation. This includes ensuring that you know of any people in your care who are at risk.

Exercise 1.25 🖉

Caring For People At Risk

Ensure the care plan explicitly states the level of supervision or observation needed for the person who is at risk. Some care plans have a necessary and appropriate element of risk which has been agreed by the care team. An example would be allowing a person to travel to the day centre without supervision when

there is a slight risk that he or she might get lost. Report any significant changes in the person's physical or mental condition immediately.

Report any signs or symptoms of abuse immediately. Sometimes it is important to point out the potential consequences of legal action that can be taken against a (potential) abuser.

Understand all legal and organisational policies and referral systems concerned with the types of abuse from which your client group are at risk. Often there are other care agencies involved when there are people at risk. Because of the implications of potential legal action, it is essential that the various agencies keep accurate records and communicate with each other.

There may be times when you learn that someone (who may or may not be a client) is at risk. Carefully explain to the person who told you that you may have to share the information with others. Where possible, the information should be checked for accuracy. If you have any concerns about dealing with abuse at work, seek advice.

Exercise 1.26 🖉

Summary

The personal characteristics that you bring to your role as a care support worker are important—personality, attitude, temperament, expectations, appearance, etc. The role requires a sincere desire to help and protect clients. Everyone deserves to be treated with respect and dignity regardless of beliefs, personal choices, race, gender, age, physical and mental abilities. Your responsibilities as a carer include promoting equality, supporting diversity, maintaining confidentiality, minimising abuse, and monitoring those at risk to ensure ethical and legal rights are upheld.

Check Your Knowledge and Understanding

1. A young mother attends a clinic for counselling with her six-month-old son. You notice that the child has a number of linear bruises to his lower back and buttocks. The mother says the bruises are a result of falls. You know the woman and suspect that the child is being abused by her common-law husband. What would you do?

   a) Immediately inform the woman that you think the child has been beaten and that you are going to inform the child protection officer.

   b) Inform the person-in-charge of the clinic about the situation.

   c) Decide to forget what you have seen on the grounds of confidentiality.

   d) Wait until you have finished work, and make an anonymous phone call to the child protection officer.

2. A person who has been a patient on your ward turns up one day. He confides that he is going to take the surgeon to court for botching his operation. He asks you to supply him with a copy of his computerised records so that they can be used as evidence in court. What would you do?

   a) Simply print a copy of the person's medical record, and give it to him.

   b) Refuse to supply him with a copy of his medical records on the grounds that patients are not allowed to see their records.

   c) Inform the nurse-in-charge, and let the nurse deal with the situation.

   d) Contact the surgeon concerned so that he or she can come down to the ward to deal with this person's request.

3. Your boss, a married man, has started sexually harassing you by making occasional lewd suggestions and telling filthy jokes. You have politely asked him to stop, but he simply replied that he was only joking and walked away. The harassment has continued. What should you do?

   a) Slap his face the next time he sexually harasses you.

   b) Ask for a transfer or look for another job.

   c) Ignore your manager in the hope that he will stop harassing you.

   d) Report your manager's behaviour to the personnel department.

4. There are times when it is appropriate to breach confidentiality. Under which of the following situations would a breach of confidentiality be appropriate?

   a) A client informs you that she is contemplating suicide.

   b) A client informs you that he has been sexually abusing his step-daughter.

   c) A good friend of a patient who has been admitted to a psychiatric unit demands to know why her friend has been admitted.

   d) An insurance company rings you to ask about the diagnosis of a patient who has recently taken out a large life insurance policy.

5. A Moslem man is admitted to your residential home. He was recently discharged from hospital after treatment for a stomach complaint where he lost a lot of weight. He needs a healthy diet, but it is Ramadan and he refuses to eat between sunrise and sunset. What would you do?

   a) Insist that he eats his special diet at the same time as the other residents.

   b) Accept his fasting, offering him a slice of toast and a cup of tea for his supper.

   c) Allow his family to leave food for you to warm up for him at the times when he is allowed to eat.

   d) Insist that he goes home if he is not willing to follow the routines of the nursing home.

6. Which of the following strategies is usually not appropriate for dealing with challenging behaviour?

   a) Getting conflicting parties to negotiate a settlement they can all live with

   b) Reprimanding a person for being abusive or aggressive

   c) Getting the conflicting parties to recommence their work

   d) Providing feedback to people about the effects of their challenging behaviour on others

7. One of the people in your care makes a complaint that a fellow resident is continually threatening him with violence. What would you do?

   a) Make an immediate written record of the details of the complaint.

   b) Write up the complaint in the care record at the end of the shift.

   c) Ignore the complaint in the hope that the situation will "cool down" over the next couple of days.

   d) Mention the problem to the person-in-charge, when she arrives on duty in four hours time.

8. Which of the following strategies is not appropriate for a person who is at slight risk of minor physical abuse.

   a) Report signs and symptoms of abuse immediately to the person-in-charge.

   b) Ensure that the care plan outlines in detail the level of supervision that is required.

   c) Keep the person under constant supervision until there is no longer a risk.

   d) Report any significant changes in the person's physical or mental condition.

Using Communication and Interpersonal Skills

Need-to-know words:

- aphasia
- articulation
- assertiveness
- communication (verbal and non-verbal)
- crisis
- interpersonal skills
- listening
- mental defence mechanism
- modulation
- rapport
- stress
- stroke
- therapeutic relationship
- unconditional positive regard

Use your communication skills to help others.

Objectives:

- Describe good communication skills.
- Identify common communication problems.
- Outline how to challenge another person's behaviour.
- Highlight barriers to communication.
- Outline how to assess communication differences.
- Assist individuals to communicate.
- Obtain and record accurate information from others.
- Manage client records according to local organisational policies.
- Transmit information to others safely and accurately.

Module 2 Introduction

Module 2 relates directly to three units of the level 2 NVQ/SVQ Award in Care:

Unit C1: **Promote effective communication and relationships** is a mandatory group A unit. It consists of two elements of competence:

- CL1.1 Develop relationships with people which value them as individuals.

- CL1.2 Establish and maintain effective communication with people.

Unit C2: **Promote communication with individuals where there are communication differences** is an option group B unit. It consists of two elements of competence:

- CL2.1 Determine the nature and scope of communication differences.

- CL2.2 Contribute to effective communication where there are communication differences.

Unit CU5: **Receive, transmit, store, and retrieve information** is also an option group B unit. It consists of two elements of competence:

- CU5.1 Receive and transmit information.

- CU5.2 Store and retrieve records.

Part 1: Developing Effective Relationships (CL1)

Everything you do or say communicates a message.

All interactions between two or more people are a form of communication. Communication occurs in many forms and has four main categories (as noted below).

	Vocal	**Non-vocal**
Verbal	Spoken word, e.g., speech, radio, television	Written word or symbol e.g., book, magazine, fax, e-mail
Non-verbal	Verbal mannerisms, e.g., sighs, stammer; vocal qualities (loudness, pitch, tone of voice)	Movement, facial expression, gestures, appearance, distance between speakers, etc.

Four Main Categories of Communication

One goal of communication is to ensure that a clear message is communicated and/or received. Other goals are to understand others and, in turn, be understood, get acceptance, and achieve effective action.

Verbal aspects of communication form an essential part of everyday life. However, people tend to have different abilities in terms of being able to interpret non-verbal aspects of communication. To recognise the information that people are trying to convey, you must try to interpret both the verbal and non-verbal aspects of communication.

Exercise 2.1 🖉

Just as a written sentence has a beginning (capital letter), a middle, and an end (full stop), all interactions between two or more people also have a form of beginning (e.g., eye contact is achieved), middle (e.g., maintaining eye contact), and end (e.g., one party breaks eye contact and walks away). People, whether or not they are from different cultures, may have different ways of, or preferences for, communicating the start, middle, and end of an interaction.

When communicating with another person, the interaction provides information about that person. Following are examples:

- Ability to communicate clearly

- Level of understanding of the issues being discussed

- Self-image that is being projected
- Mood of the person
- Aspects of personality
- Accent may indicate social class, ethnicity, or place of birth

Misinterpretation of the signals, together with prejudices, can result in your assessment of the person being very wrong. Therefore, you often need to check your initial assessment by asking the person pertinent questions (e.g., "Are you feeling anxious today, Mr. Jones?").

Exercise 2.2

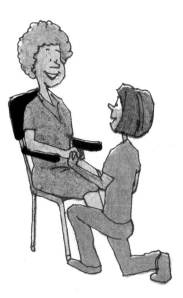

Communication generally follows culturally set rules. Most people learn the rules without being conscious of them, in the same way they do not have to think about how to walk. During good quality communication, a person plays the role of speaker and listener. *Good listeners* hear and concentrate, are attentive, and check that they understand what the speaker said. *Good speakers* use clear and concise vocabulary, provide openings (opportunities for the listener to join the conversation); use appropriate tone, pitch, and volume of voice; and use appropriate gestures and facial expressions.

Exercise 2.3

Verbal communication is only part of the message that you are trying to convey. To prevent mistakes, follow these guidelines:

- Use appropriate language when communicating with people in your care.
- Use an interpreter if you do not speak a common language. (Be aware of the impact that a third person may have on willingness to disclose and on confidentiality.)
- Communicate with people at their level of understanding. (Use an appropriate manner, level, and pace, according to individual abilities.)
- Speak slowly, repeating yourself where necessary.
- Modify your communication, if necessary, to get the message across.
- Do not shout at people who are having difficulty understanding you.
- Do not use medical jargon or long words which may be confusing.

Exercise 2.4

Non-verbal communication is at least as important as the words used in face-to-face interaction. It can replace some speech and complements the spoken word and/or reinforces what is said. It regulates the flow of communication between speaker and listener and provides feedback to the other person, thus sustaining a conversation. Non-verbal communication also defines relationships between speaker and listener and acceptable patterns of behaviour.

Many messages are conveyed by non-verbal communication. By your non-verbal actions, people can interpret whether you are happy or sad, dominant or subordinate, friendly or angry. Non-verbal behaviour varies from person to person and between cultures. Actions that are commonplace for some may be totally unacceptable to others.

Touch is less common for British people when communicating compared to the Continentals. Where you touch is bound by social rules. For example, guiding another person's movements by steering at the elbow is acceptable; putting your hand on a man's or woman's knee or thigh while talking may be highly unacceptable.

Gaze often starts an interaction. The person listening gives more eye contact than the person talking. Too much eye contact or staring creates anxiety.

Hand movements are mainly used as illustrators and emphasisers. Be aware of cultural differences. (For example, the A-OK signal made by joining the thumb and forefinger into a circle, in France, means that you are worth zero. In Italy, it describes somebody as an "asshole.") Hand movements can also replace speech (e.g., Makaton or sign language).

Facial expression is closely observed during interaction as it modifies everything that is said or done by showing emotions, providing feedback, indicating attitude, etc.

Posture is very important in communicating attitudes and feelings. For example, at the start of an informal interview, it is important to sit straight, facing the person, leaning slightly forward to indicate interest. Talk to people at the same physical level, whenever possible; standing over them can be intimidating.

Distance often indicates the relationship between two people. Spouses, lovers, and children are usually allowed within 18 inches—the "intimate" space. From 18 inches to four feet is "personal" space for friends, and four to nine feet is "social" space for most relationships. Personal space varies; what invades the personal space of one person will not do so for another.

Exercise 2.5 🖉

Listening

There are two types of listening. *Passive* listening involves the absorption of information, but the listener need not interact with the speaker (e.g., spies, eaves droppers). *Active* listening is also the absorption of information, but there is also an obvious interaction.

The active listener listens with all the senses and signals either verbally or non-verbally that the message is understood and encourages the speaker to continue.

Verbally signal active listening:

- Provide acknowledgement and confirmation of the other person (e.g., say "Yes," "Right,"

"Okay," "Mm-hmm," or make appropriate sounds where the intonation of the sounds determines the nature of the response).

- Reflect back to the person your interpretation of what was said.

- Provide appropriate praise, encouragement, and support to signal involvement on the part of the listener. The interest must appear sincere, rather than patronising.

- Appropriately interrupt or disagree to stimulate interaction (not in a way that communicates that you think what you have to say is more important).

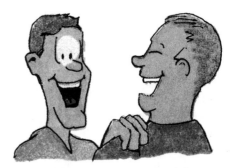

Non-verbally signal active listening:

- Indicate with the head (e.g., nods) and facial expressions (e.g., smiles, frowns).
- Use appropriate eye contact.
- Mirror similar facial expressions and body position.
- Adopt an attentive posture.

Exercise 2.6 🖉

General Barriers to Communication

Barriers to communication affect relationships and interfere with interaction. Avoid the following barriers:

- Appearing bored or impatient
- Threatening others or using harsh language
- Jumping to conclusions
- Negating, devaluing, or being critical of others
- Mumbling or confused presentation

- Arguing or interrupting
- Ignoring
- Passing judgment or giving unwanted advice
- Confusing people with multiple questions
- Distracting (e.g., fiddling or doodling)
- Having physical barriers between you and the client (e.g., a desk)
- Being in environments that are distracting or uncomfortable

Enhancing Relationships

Good relationships are the foundation of a comfortable working experience. Treating people with respect and dignity builds good relationships.

Always knock before entering a person's room. Remember that this is an individual's living quarters. Provide the privacy and courtesy you would show to people in their own homes.

Introduce yourself. Some people have difficulty remembering names. Say your name whenever you enter a person's room to avoid confusion or embarrassment.

Ask how a person wishes to be addressed. Some people prefer not to be called by their first names.

Provide comfort. Pay attention to each person's needs.

Support individual rights and choices within the limits of your work role. Encourage individuals to express their wishes and needs.

Be courteous and respectful of visitors. Family and friends influence the well-being of clients. Provide privacy if desired. If you must provide care, politely ask visitors to leave the room, and let them know when they can return.

Maintain privacy and dignity at all times. Everyone wants to be loved and have friends with shared interests. Regardless of age, people are sexual beings with sexual desires. Deal with sexuality in a mature, professional manner. Allow privacy, and do not interfere with consenting partners as long as the individuals concerned are not likely to come to any harm. If problems arise, ask your manager how to handle the situation.

Exercise 2.7

Challenging Unacceptable Behaviour

Remember that different people behave differently and can have very different views on the acceptability of behaviour. This will depend on a person's attitude and values which have been moulded by upbringing and life experiences. One person's appropriate and acceptable behaviour may be unreasonable and offensive to another person (e.g., somebody is offended by another person's rude or warped sense of humour).

The crux of the matter comes when you feel that someone has overstepped the mark of acceptable behaviour. In some cases, it is appropriate to challenge the person (e.g., when somebody makes repeated sexist remarks to you, or when someone's behaviour is upsetting the people in your care). The challenge can take the form of a gentle reminder of more appropriate ways to behave, or you may need to be assertive in your challenge.

At other times, you can appropriately laugh off or ignore another person's undesirable behaviour (e.g., when someone accidentally spills a drink and swears). Remember to take into account the cultural norms for the situation, and try to balance them against your personal beliefs.

Exercise 2.8

The following examples are assertive ways that you can choose to challenge another person's behaviour:

- Say, "I find swearing offensive; please do not swear in front of me again."

- Remind the person that the behaviour is upsetting and/or offending other people.

- Inform the person that the behaviour is illegal (e.g., racist, sexist, or likely to cause a breach of the peace) and that you will inform your manager/the police if the behaviour does not stop.

Choose the correct time and place to challenge another person's behaviour, or you may make the situation worse. The person may not be able to stop behaving this way (e.g., due to mental illness, epilepsy, dementia, intoxication). In these situations, choosing ways other than directly challenging the person are usually more effective at managing the situation.

Part 2: Overcoming Communication Differences (CL2)

Promote communication for people who have communication difficulties.

The model on the right, explains differences in the ways that people communicate. Messages are taken in by the body's senses (e.g., sight, hearing, touch, and smell). These are then decoded so that the person can interpret an initial meaning. In turn, they are transferred to other parts of the brain where they are linked with a person's ideas, feelings, values, and attitudes so that the message is fully understood.

When messages are to be sent out, a person's ideas, feelings, values, and attitude affect that person's intention and eventual behaviour selection. This is encoded into a message that is suitable for transmission before the message is given out by the person (via a variety of modes of communication—verbal and non-verbal).

Most aspects of taking in and sending out messages are automatic; that is, you do not have to think about it to be able to do it. It takes energy to actively listen for messages and concentrate on giving out a correct message. To communicate effectively, four basics are necessary:

- Good physical and mental health

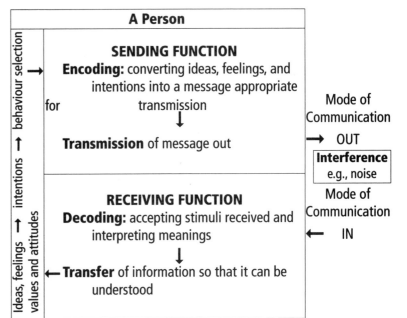

Model of Communication

- A common language

- Normal physical and psychological development through childhood to the present time

- A minimum of communication interference in the environment

Exercise 2.9 ✎

Specific Barriers to Communication

People vary in intelligence, education, religion, culture, social background, and experience. These differences create very different frames of reference where each person sees the world in a different and unique way.

All the areas outlined in the communication model on the previous page can be the focus for barriers to communication. Specific barriers to communication are outlined below.

Environmental interference: Noise may make it difficult to hear and be heard. Distractions such as bright sunlight, several people speaking at once, smells, dress, and appearance of others can interfere with communication. Level of comfort including too hot or cold, discomfort (e.g., shoes rubbing), and lack of privacy can also interfere.

Decoding barriers: Sensory problems such as poor sight or hearing affect communication. Other barriers include the language used and accent (e.g., Geordie, French, sign language), terminology, and unfamiliar words. Level of attention and any preoccupations (e.g., with catching the train home) are also barriers, as well as length of communication, memory, and ability to discriminate.

Comprehension barriers: Mental health problems (e.g., thought blocking), low intelligence, inability to comprehend, and level of knowledge about the subject area being discussed are barriers to communication. Other barriers include attitudes and values, stereotypes, and prejudices, level of anxiety and worry, mental defence mechanisms, strong emotions, and verbal and non-verbal messages not matching.

Encoding barriers: Mental health problems (i.e., confusion and disorientation) and low intelligence affect communication. Concentrating on yourself (i.e., deciding that you are going to get your message across, no matter what) also affects communication.

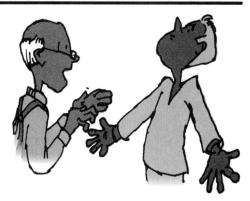

Other barriers include level of knowledge about the subject area being discussed, attitudes and values, stereotypes and prejudices, level of anxiety and worry, strong emotions, and unwillingness to communicate or tell the truth.

Transmission barriers: Physical problems (e.g., limb paralysis, inability to articulate properly, sore throat) can affect communication. Other barriers include language and accent used (e.g., French, sign language), terminology and unfamiliar words, level of attention and any preoccupations (e.g., concerned about making a mistake), and length of communication and memory.

Ensure that other professionals are used, where appropriate, to assess communication problems and overcome communication differences (e.g., speech therapist, interpreter, psychologist).

Exercise 2.10 ✎

Barriers to communication can interfere with the provision of quality care. The following examples can be the result of poor communication:

- Non-compliance with the requests of care staff
- Misunderstandings that lead to lack of trust
- Distress caused by not being able to communicate well
- Reduction in a person's self-esteem
- Difficulty in assessing other problems
- Confusion leading to mistakes being made
- Anger, depression, and feelings of helplessness when care needs are not met

Assessing Communication Differences

To accurately assess communication problems, there is a need to develop a rapport. The best way to build a rapport is by generating empathy with the other person. This involves listening to what the other person has to say and, more importantly, watching the person's response. While a person may say how he or she is feeling, non-verbal communication provides clues to how the person is really feeling.

Assessing communication problems can be difficult because of the time needed to carry out an accurate assessment. Care workers often have many people that require their care, limiting the amount of time that can be spent with one person. The time is further limited by other activities (e.g., the need to keep accurate records, answering the telephone).

It is often appropriate to seek further information about a person's communication abilities by approaching other sources (e.g., family, friends, other professionals). This can help to determine the correct method of communication to use. Sometimes a person is known to have good communication skills, but simply chooses not to use them. Or the situation may prevent the person from using good communication skills.

Communication skills are usually assessed in more detail after a communication problem has been identified by the care staff. Detailed assessments are usually carried out by a speech therapist. The only time communication skills assessments are carried out by care staff is when they are part of a larger assessment of a person's general abilities or level of development. (Examples include Portage checklist for the assessment of a child's level of development, and Progress Assessment Chart for the assessment of the abilities of people who have learning disabilities.)

Exercise 2.11 🖊

Assisting Individuals to Communicate

Before planning commences, the level and type of assistance needed by the individual should be established by assessment. Care strategies should be appropriate to the person's level of understanding and preferred mode of communication. The carer should try to use both verbal and non-verbal skills, as appropriate, that are consistent with the person's own expression and use. Preferably, different methods of overcoming the communication problem should be identified in the care plan. Aids to communication should be made available where appropriate (e.g., notepad and pencil, computer, flashcards).

The communication used by care staff should be consistent with the plan of care and delivered at an appropriate pace and level of understanding. Create opportunities for the person to communicate (e.g., during leisure activities and while care is being provided). Encourage, stimulate, and interest the person in order to promote communication. Remember that a person's communication abilities may not be indicative of the person's level of understanding.

When the plan of care includes recording of the person's communication skills, be clear, concise, and objective. Be aware of the times when the person, appropriately, may not want to communicate. Be aware of and sensitive to any conflicts between the care plan and the person's choice of communication. (For example, the plan of care might be to stimulate the person to speak, but the person might be too embarrassed to demonstrate a speech impediment.)

Be aware that there are many different ways to overcome communication difficulties and differences. Following are examples of ways to enhance communication:

- Identify yourself when entering the room, and explain what you are going to do.
- Be clear about what you want to say, and choose an appropriate time.
- Be patient.
- Carefully choose the location, and provide privacy as needed.
- Use communication aids (e.g., pictures, paper and pencil).

- Ensure that the person can clearly see your face, especially if he or she reads lips.

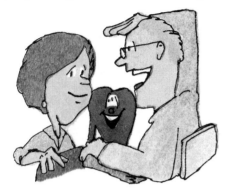

- Get close to the person who is partially deaf, and speak loudly enough to be heard without shouting (speaking to the side where hearing is best).
- Eliminate unnecessary noises (e.g., TV, radio).
- Address the person by name.
- Speak slowly; use simple words and appropriate language.
- Make the message clear, without too many details.
- Take time to check that the person understands you.
- Allow time for the person to respond.
- Use "touch" as appropriate.
- Modify a message so that it can be understood (e.g., giving examples, providing an analogy, using pictures, emphasizing facial expressions and tone of voice).
- Be supportive and positive.
- Remember that concepts are often difficult to translate into other languages (including sign language).
- Talk normally; do not "talk down" to the person nor shout.
- Ask the person to repeat if necessary, rather than pretending to understand.
- If the person uses a hearing aid, make sure that it is being worn and that it is clean.

- Use gestures when appropriate.
- Remind anyone who needs spectacles to wear them, and offer to clean the spectacles if necessary.

Exercise 2.12 🖉

Sensory Aids

Sensory aids contribute to people's well-being and independence. They help people to rely more on themselves and less on others. Encourage clients to use their sensory aids. Ensure that clients know how to use their devices. Keep devices clean and make sure that they are in good condition, if clients are not able to do this for themselves.

Hearing Aids

Hearing aids require special care. Be cautious when handling them because they are fragile. Avoid accidentally dropping them by using a table or desk for cleaning or changing batteries.

Keep hearing aids dry, as water and damp ruins them. Remove hearing aids before showering or swimming. If the aid gets wet, dry it with a soft cloth; never use heat.

Keep hearing aids clean. Use a soft cloth for cleaning them. Never use water, alcohol, cleaning solvents, oil, or sharp instruments (e.g., paper clips, pen knives). Remove aids before using hair spray.

Extend the life of batteries, as they are expensive. Turn off the hearing aid when not in use. Disconnect the battery contact for storage during the night, and remove the battery if the hearing aid is not to be used for more than 24 hours. Check to ensure that the battery is working before placing the device in a person's ear.

Store hearing aids in a safe place. Always use a case for storing the hearing aid, and mark the case with the person's name. Never leave the hearing aid where children can play with it. Discourage clients from putting hearing aids in their pockets as the aids may get sent to the laundry with clothing.

Problem	Possible Cause	Action
Doesn't Work	dead battery, plugged ear mould	replace battery, clean ear mould
Not Loud Enough	low battery, plugged ear mould, hearing may have changed	replace battery, clean ear mould, have hearing checked
Distorted	low battery	replace battery
Fuzzy	faulty hearing aid	check with supplier
Goes On and Off	bad battery, faulty hearing aid	replace battery, check with supplier
Causes Discomfort	improperly placed, wrong style	check placement, check with supplier

Common Problems with Hearing Aids

The chart above provides basic information for common problems with hearing aids and easy actions to resolve the problems.

Exercise 2.13

Spectacles

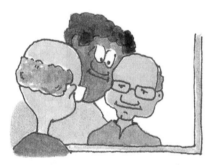

Encourage people who need spectacles to wear them. Protect the spectacles from loss or damage, since they are often misplaced and easily broken. Provide a neck strap to keep the spectacles within reach, and ensure that there is a case for storing them. For easy identification, engrave the person's name on the inside of the frame.

Clean spectacles with a soft cloth; paper tissue can scratch plastic lenses. Check them regularly for loose or missing screws and nose pieces.

Alternative Communication

Some people have severe disabilities which force them to use alternative modes of communication. Following are some examples.

Packs of flashcards highlight a commonly used word (e.g., toilet) on each card. When the person wants to communicate, a card is simply held up.

Communication boards feature a series of pictures in squares to which the person can point in order to communicate.

Computers are often provided for people with the most severe communication disabilities. The computer can be operated by various means (e.g., a blowpipe, pointer attached to the forehead, eye movements, keyboard, mouse).

Various other methods of communication are available to support individuals who have communication difficulties (e.g., Makaton, British Sign Language, Amerind).

Makaton is a language programme which has two vocabularies. The first is a small core vocabulary of essential words required for everyday conversational needs. The second is a much broader vocabulary which covers a wide range of life experiences. These two vocabularies are used, when possible, with speech, British Sign Language, and Makaton symbols. Many of the signs resemble the activity or object that the words are intended to symbolise. The system makes it possible for people who have difficulty with fine movements to make a satisfactory attempt at communication using the signs.

The Makaton core vocabulary consists of a special selection of the most essential and useful words for basic everyday communication. It is structured in stages of increasing complexity. Initial stages include a basic vocabulary to express essential needs. Subsequent stages expand the range of signs so that more complex language can be used.

Only the key words are signed, but signs should always be accompanied by normal speech. Where appropriate, use facial expressions with the signs, especially when conveying emotions. There are no strict rules regarding the precise performance of the signs (e.g., size and distance from body).

If you provide care for a person who uses Makaton, try to learn the core vocabulary. Gain some knowledge of the symbols and how to use Makaton with people who have communication and/or learning difficulties.

Exercise 2.14

Part 3: Managing Information (CU5)

Carefully manage information according to local policies.

An important part of your role is the management of records and information. If you have any worries or uncertainties about managing information, seek advice from your manager or an appropriately experienced colleague (e.g., IT manager, data protection officer).

Information is available in many formats nowadays—paper-based (e.g., books, leaflets, publications, charts, faxes), electronic (e.g., compact discs, computer e-mail, network databases), and verbal (e.g., television, radio, speech).

Exercise 2.15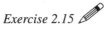

Obtaining Information

Information about clients and the care services that they are receiving often needs to be obtained from clients, their families, friends, and other care workers. Ensure that your request for information is appropriate, and be clear about the information you need. Specify the timescale within which you need the information, and allow time for the person to respond. When necessary, confirm the relevance and accuracy of the information that you are given. Check that the information is up-to-date, and seek further information, if required.

If the information that is being obtained is of a personal nature, ensure that this information can be obtained in private. If necessary, signal to colleagues (verbally or non-verbally) to leave the area/room while the information is being given to you. Always safeguard confidential information. (See the principles of the Data Protection Act, 1998, in Module 1.)

Gathering information requires varying degrees of detail. For example, if a person is being admitted to a care establishment, you may have to collect personal details such as name, address, date of birth, etc. If the person cannot provide details of non-essential information at the time of admission, these details can be obtained later (e.g., when a client forgets his postcode).

Be thorough when collecting information. It is important that you check for accuracy, currency, and relevancy to the situation. For example, if the information pertains to child abuse, it may be needed for use in court. Also, it is no good sending an appointment to an address if the person no longer lives there.

Another example is when a patient is sent to the operating theatre. The patient wears a wrist band for identification that contains his or her hospital number. The band is checked prior to leaving the surgical ward and again against the operating list after entering the operating theatre. This ensures that the patient is not given the wrong operation.

Observing

Being a skilled observer helps to identify and prevent serious problems from occurring and earns the respect of your colleagues. Being alert to people and their environment helps to reduce accidents and maintains the well-being of the people in your care.

Exercise 2.16

Careful observation increases your awareness of each person's physical, emotional, and social needs. Learn to recognise the signs and symptoms of common diseases and conditions. One of the major keys to helping clients is to detect problems in their early stages.

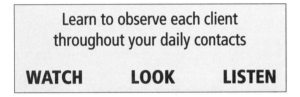

Learn to observe each client throughout your daily contacts
WATCH   **LOOK**   **LISTEN**

Trust your instincts. If something appears to be wrong, report it. Any physical or emotional change may indicate a deterioration or improvement in the health and well-being of the client.

Be alert to physical changes:

• Odour	• Spasms
• Blurred vision	• Excessive thirst
• Swelling, oedema	• Nausea, vomiting
• Rash, hives, blisters	• Cold, pale, clammy
• Ringing in the ears	• Drowsiness, lethargy
• Pain, difficulty, discomfort	• Hot, sweating, burning, feverish
• Diarrhoea, constipation	• Choking, coughing, wheezing, sneezing

- Abnormally decreased increased body functions (e.g., elimination, pulse, breathing)
- Unconsciousness, or weakness, dizziness, trembling

Be alert to emotional changes:

- Mood swings
- Depressed, feelings of helplessness and hopelessness, crying, tearful
- Angry, difficult, irrational
- Disoriented, confused
- Anxious, frightened, pacing

Exercise 2.17

Managing Records

Records are important documents that can be in the form of paperwork or electronic data. Before you start, complete, or update a record, make sure that you have the correct record. Be careful to enter only accurate data. Inaccurate data entries can be illegal and dangerous.

Ensure that you store records safely so that the records can be retrieved and used in the future. Make a note when records are transferred to other locations, and ensure that you know where they have been sent so that they can be traced, if necessary. The records must be safely and securely stored/locked away when not in use. Confidential records held on computer should be guarded by an access code so that only those people who know the access code can gain access to the information.

Make sure that you know your organisation's policies relating to confidentiality, access, and transmission of information pertaining to your role. This includes knowing the records that can be accessed by people receiving care, and those to which they should not have access. For example, it is appropriate that a person should have access to his or her own medical records, but not to budget sheets or the accident book for a particular organisation.

Inform your manager if your part of the organisation maintains, stores, and retrieves records in a way that conflicts with good practice. For example, in a busy department, it is easy to leave confidential records lying around where they can be illegally accessed.

Making Records

Accuracy is very important. A person's health record is a legal document. It is often used as a diagnostic aid and to judge how an illness or problem is responding to treatment or problem management. Follow these guidelines when updating a person's record:

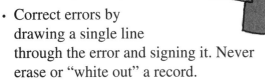

- Write notes on a spare piece of paper first, and then check for accuracy and spelling.

- Write clearly and neatly in ink (preferably black, unless otherwise indicated, as specified in organisational policies).

- Correct errors by drawing a single line through the error and signing it. Never erase or "white out" a record.

- Always date and time your record, as appropriate.

- Chart only the procedures that you have done, after they have been done, at the earliest opportunity.

- Chart reports of your observations.

- Always sign your entries.

- Make sure that you maintain the confidentiality of all chart/record entries.

Exercise 2.18

Reporting

All care workers require ongoing information (e.g., end-of-shift reports, staff meeting reports). This information is required for the ongoing assessment and planning that is required to meet client needs so that high quality care can be provided. Accurate reports about a person's condition, problems, or needs are made to the supervisor as often as required. End-of-shift reports to the staff coming on duty provide the information necessary for continuity of care. Each client report should include the individual's name and a detailed outline of all the relevant factors about that client's care.

Objective reporting is precisely what you can physically see, hear, smell, or feel. If a person complains of symptoms that you cannot observe, such as dizziness or pain, report exactly what the client says to you.

Correct: Mrs. Smith says her left ear aches.

Correct: Mr. Jones' right arm is red, swollen, and warm to the touch.

Subjective reporting is used to report what you cannot sense. Where possible, avoid subjective reporting. However, if you think that something is wrong, medically or emotionally, or if the client complains of a problem, report it to your supervisor and make a record of it, if appropriate.

Incorrect: Mrs. Smith has an ear infection.

Correct: Mrs. Smith is holding her left ear and she appears to be in some discomfort.

Exercise 2.19

Transmitting Information

The transmission of information to others is an essential component of quality care. Accurate information is necessary in order to avoid mistakes and misunderstandings.

Before giving out information, politely check the enquirer's identity (preferably by looking at the person's

ID card/badge), and check that the person has the authority to access the information. If a person has the right of access, but you do not have the required information to hand, inform the person when you can provide the information, or refer the person to someone who can meet his or her needs. Since identity cannot be checked over the telephone, never provide confidential information over the telephone.

Messages

Ask callers to write down and leave their own messages, where possible. If this is not possible (e.g., the person is in a hurry), write down the message immediately so that you do not forget it. Use the prescribed message slips, if available. Read your written message to the person to check for accuracy and clarity.

All telephone messages should be written down. Write the message during the phone call or immediately afterwards so that you do not forget the details. Before hanging up, read the message back to the person to check for accuracy and clarity.

If you receive messages for others that have been sent by fax or e-mail, provide a paper copy of the message to the recipient at the earliest opportunity. Or, you may be required to transmit the message by fax, e-mail, telephone, or face-to-face. If the message is unclear or indistinct, you may have to contact the sender to either resend the message or provide clarification. If required, ask the recipient of the message to contact you to confirm the message was received.

All messages should include the name of the person sending the message and the name of the person who is to receive the message, plus the signature of the person passing on the message. Include the date and time the message was received and the date and time the message was given to the person. Ensure that details of the message are clear, and indicate whether it is urgent. Add whether it was a verbal or telephone message. If the message is confidential, this should be clearly indicated on the message sheet.

Exercise 2.20

Choose an appropriate method to transmit the message, and get the information to the intended person within a "reasonable" time, depending on the urgency of the message. You may need to disturb a person in a meeting if the message is urgent. If in doubt about the urgency of a message, seek advice.

Check the identity of the person to whom you are delivering the message. If necessary, explain the message so that the person understands what it means. If you hand the message to another person for delivery, ensure that the person understands the urgency of the message. Make sure the message is in an envelope marked "confidential" if it contains confidential information.

If you are delivering the message over the telephone and the person is not available, do not leave a message if you are concerned about confidentiality. Simply leave your name and telephone number so that the person can contact you. Before sending a message by fax, consider whether that would be appropriate, especially if the fax machine to which you are sending it is where it can be seen by passers-by.

If the message is important, but not confidential (e.g., a change of venue for a meeting that day), and you do not know where the intended recipient is located, you may want to saturate all possible locations (e.g., send an e-mail, leave a telephone message, and/or send a fax to each possible location).

Exercise 2.21

Summary

Everything you do and say communicates a message, and the ability to communicate well builds good relationships. Choose your words carefully, and reflect a caring attitude with your listening skills, facial expressions, gestures, posture, etc. As a carer, you need to deal effectively with unacceptable behaviour and to overcome communication differences. Understanding stress helps you to prevent and manage stress in the care environment and to support clients in times of distress. Take care to manage client information according to local policies.

Check Your Knowledge and Understanding

1. Which of the following are communication problems?

   a) A person speaks a foreign language that you do not understand.

   b) A person is not telling the truth.

   c) A person has misinterpreted what you have said.

   d) A person is distressed and angry.

2. A person in your care is a little confused, and she is to be discharged home this afternoon. She needs to know about the medication that has been prescribed for her to take home. She also needs to know about the place that has been organised for her at a day centre. What would you do?

   a) Inform the lady about her discharge plan, and hope that she understands and remembers the information.

   b) Inform the lady, and then write the information down on a sheet of paper for her to keep as a reminder.

   c) Do not inform the lady. Inform the relative who will soon arrive to take her home.

   d) Inform both the lady and the relative, and provide them with the sheet of paper that has all the details.

3. In planning care to overcome a communication difference or problem, which of the following is/are incorrect?

   a) A full assessment of the communication problem should be carried out before the care is planned.

   b) The person should be asked to speak plain English.

   c) You should try to encourage a distressed person, who is not yet ready to talk, to discuss potential answers to his personal problems.

   d) Preferably, different methods for overcoming the communication problem should be identified in the care plan.

4. One of your residents in a care home insists on telling crude jokes and attempts to pinch the bottoms of carers whenever he gets the opportunity. His behaviour is making some of the carers avoid him, and he is upsetting some of the other residents. What should you do?

   a) Reprimand the resident, informing him that he will be asked to leave if he misbehaves again.

   b) Ignore his behaviour in the hope that it will stop.

   c) Move him to a side ward where the other residents will not be bothered by his behaviour. Leave a note in the office reminding carers not to bend down in front of him.

   d) Have a quiet word with him. Describe the effects that his sexual assaults and jokes are having on the carers and the other residents. Negotiate with him to stop pinching bottoms and to "tone down" his jokes.

5. You notice that Jane, a person in your care, has severe abrasions to the outside of her left arm. She refuses to tell you how it happened. Jane has a past history of self-injury, including scraping her arms against the wall while walking down the street. What would be the most accurate way that you could report this in her care record?

a) "Jane has been scraping her arm along the wall again, resulting in some severe abrasions to her left arm."

b) "Jane has severe abrasions on her left arm. It looks as though she has started injuring herself again."

c) "Jane has severe abrasions on her left arm. She refuses to say how this happened."

d) "Jane has hurt her left arm. It is not known how this happened."

6. You are using your organisation's computer database to access a client record for a forthcoming case conference. Your access code does not allow you entry to a relevant report on this client from a child protection officer. What would you do?

a) Ask a colleague to access the computer's hard disk to try and bypass the computer's security protection on the child protection report.

b) Ask to borrow a colleague's access code so that you can download a copy of the report that you need.

c) Contact the child protection officer, and ask her to fax or e-mail the report to you or send a copy through the post.

d) Inform your manager that you cannot access the child protection report. Someone else will have to access that report if it is to be available for the case conference.

7. A message comes through to your office that a colleague's daughter has been injured at school and admitted to hospital. Your colleague will be in a case conference for the next hour or more. What would you do?

a) Write a message for your colleague on the white board so that she will see it when she leaves the case conference.

b) Interrupt the case conference immediately, and ask your colleague to come out of the meeting so that you can give her the message.

c) Write out the message, and leave it on your colleague's desk or her in-tray.

d) Inform your colleague as soon as she leaves the case conference.

8. An elderly and disabled lady who lives alone in the community phones to inform the community nurse that she has run out of her tranquilliser tablets. The nurse is out on her rounds and will be returning at lunch time. What should you do?

a) Write the message on a message slip, and leave it on the nurse's desk.

b) Try to contact the nurse immediately by phoning all the patients that she is due to visit that morning.

c) Verbally pass on the message to the nurse when she arrives at lunch time, if you see her.

d) Pass the message on to one of the nurse's colleagues so that she can deliver it.

9. A "social worker" arrives at a residential home, wanting to interview one of the residents and have access to one of the resident's case notes. Nobody at the home has seen this social worker before, and he carries no identification. What would you do?

a) Accept the social worker's word and allow him access to the resident and the case notes.

b) Tell the social worker to go away and not come back until he has found his ID card.

c) Phone the social work department and ask for a description of the social worker to confirm his identity.

d) Allow the social worker access to the resident, but not to the case notes. Then make a formal complaint to the social work department about the social worker not carrying an ID card.

Module 3

Providing Ongoing Support

Support clients and others significant to them.

Objectives:

- Outline the reasons why an individual may not be able to take part in leisure pursuits.
- Highlight how to enable others to take part in leisure pursuits.
- Outline the reasons why a client may not be able to keep in contact with significant others.
- Describe how to enable a client to keep in contact with significant others.
- Outline the preparation and support that are required for visits between clients and significant others.
- Highlight how carers can support clients.
- Describe how to enable a carer to provide health care for a client.
- List the reasons why a change of care environment for a client may be necessary.
- Outline the preparation and support that are required when a client's care environment is changed.

Module 3 Introduction

Module 3 relates to two units of the level 2 NVQ/SVQ Award in Care:

Unit W2: **Contribute to the ongoing support of clients and others significant to them** is an option group B unit. It consists of four elements of competence:

- W2.1 Enable clients to maintain their interests, identity, and emotional well-being whilst receiving care services.

- W2.2 Enable clients to maintain contact with those who are significant to them.

- W2.3 Support those who are significant to clients, during visits.

- W2.4 Enable carers to support clients.

Unit W3: **Support individuals experiencing a change in their care requirements and provision** is an option group B unit. It consists of two elements of competence:

- W3.1 Enable individuals to prepare for, and transfer to, different care environments.

- W3.2 Enable individuals to become familiar with new care requirements.

Part 1: Contributing to Ongoing Support (W2)

Enable clients to maintain their interests, well-being, and relationships.

Clients and their significant others (e.g., spouse, relatives, friends) need a wide variety of ongoing support services from the care worker. The type of support will depend on the client's general health and well-being, the type of care services required by the client, the limitations imposed by the care environment, and the care roles that can be undertaken by the client and significant others.

The aim of providing support to clients and significant others is to ensure that their experiences of ongoing support and care for the client's illness or disability can be viewed as a developmental and beneficial process.

Leisure pursuits can help to maintain an individual's physical and psychological well-being, personal identity, and self-esteem. Activities prevent boredom and help to reduce the stresses of everyday life. Benefits include fitness, flexibility, dexterity, and mental alertness.

Most people have at least one hobby, interest, or pastime that they enjoy doing on a regular basis. An individual's choice of leisure pursuits will depend on a number of factors such as personal preference, cultural and family norms and expectations, health and level of fitness, and the resources available to the individual. Where appropriate, it is important that clients continue their leisure pursuits, or resume them at the earliest opportunity.

Exercise 3.1 🖉

Leisure pursuits can be **sedentary** or **non-sedentary**. Following are examples of *sedentary* activities:

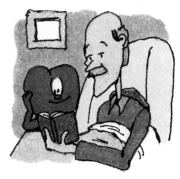

- Reading
- Knitting/crocheting
- Watching sports
- Visiting the pub
- Doing crafts
- Using the computer
- Listening to music
- Watching television
- Playing board and card games

Following are examples of *non-sedentary* activities:

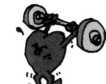

- Exercising
- Walking
- Gardening
- Dancing
- Participating in active sports (e.g., football, netball)
- Doing handicrafts (e.g., wood work, decorating)

All non-sedentary activities involve varying amounts of physical activity. However, sedentary activities involve very little or no physical activity

Exercise 3.2 ✎

A number of problems can prevent an individual from taking part in leisure pursuits. Following are examples:

- **Physical illness** (e.g., an individual with a broken leg would not be able to play football; an individual with vision problems would have difficulty playing darts or sewing)

- **Mental health problems** (e.g., an individual who suffers from claustrophobia may find it difficult to be in crowds; an individual who has anxiety attacks may find it very difficult to take part in highly competitive team games)

- **Disability** (e.g., an individual who has colitis may find it difficult to take part in cross-country walks because of the need for regular access to a toilet; an individual who develops dementia would find it difficult to continue to play chess)

- **Environmental problems** (e.g., an individual who enjoys going to the cinema in the city, but lives at a residential home in a village that only has two buses per day; a young woman who is not able to go walking alone locally because it is a very rough neighbourhood where she may be at risk of being attacked)

- **Financial problems** (e.g. redundancy and the subsequent loss of income resulting in having to relinquish membership of the local golf club; not being able to afford wool for knitting)

As with any other client problem, a thorough assessment of the situation needs to be undertaken. The emphasis is on meeting the client's needs for relaxation and/or diversionary activities. Until you find out precisely what is going to meet the client's needs in the short- and long-term, you cannot plan to meet those needs. Take care to ensure that you do not stereotype a client as a particular type with particular interests.

Five approaches can be used to manage the situation when people are unable to take part in their usual leisure pursuits.

Discontinue the activity, and enable the individual to **restart** at the earliest possible opportunity. (This approach is usually only acceptable in the short-term.)

Discontinue the activity, and **divert** the person into another activity (e.g., a person who has been made redundant cannot afford to play golf, may be happy to take up cross-country walking to keep fit).

Access the resources necessary to enable the individual to take part in the leisure activity (e.g., welfare benefits may be available for undertaking leisure pursuits that are necessary for health and well-being).

Adapt the activity (e.g., an individual who is having problems sewing because of a vision problem can be provided with a vision aid such as a large magnifying lens, special glasses, or modified equipment such as large needles and a needle threader).

Convert the activity from non-sedentary to sedentary (e.g., a person with a broken leg cannot continue to play football, but could go to see the team's matches during the recovery period).

Exercise 3.3 ✎

Promoting Leisure Pursuits

Acceptance of a client's leisure pursuits is part of accepting the client as a person. Even when you feel that a client's interests are rather boring or bizarre, support the client in undertaking them, as long as the leisure pursuits are safe, affordable, legal, and compatible with the overall plan of care.

Always provide clients with the opportunity to express their own views concerning the support they think is appropriate to enable them to undertake their chosen leisure pursuit(s). Flexible assistance, support, and companionship should be provided in a way which meets the clients' changing needs, as long as it is compatible with the plan of care and your care role.

Clients should be encouraged to be as independent as possible in following their chosen leisure pursuits. Where appropriate, ensure that colleagues are aware of clients' leisure pursuits and that they are part of the plan of care, especially when advice, support, guidance, or a physical presence is necessary.

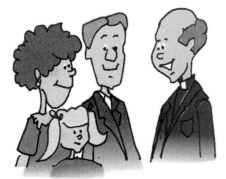

Significant Others

Significant others can be partners, relatives, friends, religious leaders, and even pets. Most people have a range of significant others with whom they would like to keep in contact, even when receiving care. Maintaining contacts with significant others is very important for children as they can have a significant effect on their emotional and intellectual development, especially in terms of bonding and attachment.

Exercise 3.4 🖋

Acceptance of a client's significant others and the client's need to maintain or avoid contact with them is important. Even when you feel that contact with specific individuals may not be in the client's best interest, support the client, as long as the contacts are safe (e.g., not likely to result in significant danger or abuse to the client or others), affordable (e.g., telephone bills), and compatible with the overall plan of care.

Where appropriate, ensure that colleagues are aware of clients' contacts with significant others and that they are part of the plan of care, especially when advice, support, guidance, or a physical presence is required by the client and/or significant others.

Always provide the opportunity for clients to express their own views in relation to significant others with whom they would like to keep in contact. Provide the support they think is appropriate to enable them to maintain the contacts. Be flexible in meeting the client's changing needs, as long as it is compatible with the plan of care and your care role. Encourage clients to be as independent as possible in maintaining contacts with significant others.

Communication with significant others vary in degrees of contact/intimacy. Communication includes:

- Face-to-face visits
- Correspondence (letters and postcards)
- Using the Internet
- Telephone calls

The forms of communication that are used by a client will depend on the person's physical and mental abilities, the preferred ways of communicating with others, and the finances and physical resources (equipment) that are available (e.g., telephone, fax, computer, communication boards). An outline of the main aspects of communication can be seen in Module 2.

Exercise 3.5 🖋

When visits occur infrequently or not at all, communications between clients and significant others

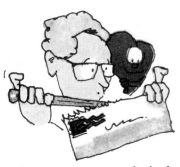

can be very important. Messages should be delivered promptly, accurately, completely and confidentially. When a client wishes you to correspond with, or contact, another person on their behalf, ensure that you communicate with the other person using the mode of communication preferred by the client (e.g., verbal message, letter). Also, communicate accurately and legibly, in a way which clearly reflects the client's intended message. Let the client check the message or letter before it is sent.

Information about the client is only divulged to those people who have a right to know (e.g., spouse, partner, or close relative). The main exception here is when the client has indicated that specific individuals are not to receive information about him or her. (See Module 2 for guidelines on confidentiality.) If you have worries about communications between a client and another person (e.g., a relative sends an abusive letter, a client is asking a person to send drugs), report your worries to the person-in-charge.

Exercise 3.6

Visits

Visits to significant others involve clients in travelling to meet them at their homes, or in places other than their own homes. Visits usually need to be planned. It is important that all relevant care staff are aware of an individual's care plan relating to client visits. This can be important during the planning of the visit, especially when you or others may need to provide assistance with making the arrangements and preparing for the visit in a manner that meets the client's needs and wishes.

For visits to others, ensure that arrangements have been made with the person who is to be visited so that the date, time, and venue for the visit are agreed. Arrange for the type and timing of transport to and from the venue for the client and, if necessary, an escort. Consider the level of support, if any, that is required during the visit.

Where appropriate, ensure that the client is properly dressed for the visit. Take a pair of Wellington boots if a muddy walk is anticipated, and take a coat (evenings may be cold, even on the warmest days). If required, ensure that the client remembers to keep any money safe and that he or she takes along any necessary medication.

The care team may need to do a risk assessment if the client or others could be placed in danger by the visit. This may require certain restrictions for the purposes of meeting legal requirements (e.g., a care worker is always to be present during the visit) or health care needs (e.g., specified medical equipment must accompany the client at all times).

Exercise 3.7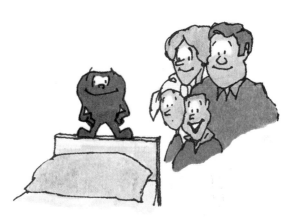

To prepare for visitors, arrangements may have to be made with the person who is visiting so that the date, time, and venue for the visit are agreed. Some care environments may have restrictions on visiting (e.g., rest periods for clients). Visitors may need advice in terms of directions to the venue, the forms of public transport that are available, and/or the availability of parking. Arrangements may need to be made so that visitors are politely greeted, made to feel at ease, and directed or escorted to the place where the visit is to take place.

The client and visitors may need to be advised regarding any legal restrictions on their freedom of movement and level of supervision during the visit. According to the client's wishes, arrangements may need to be made to ensure that as much privacy as possible is provided during the visit (e.g., separate room, curtained bed space, cordoned off cubicle, a quiet corner). Consider the level of support, if any, that is required by the client and visitors during the visit.

Exercise 3.8 🖉

During visits, depending on the level of support that is required, your role may include providing psychological support (especially if the visit is likely to be stressful), physical support in terms of helping the person to mobilise, ensuring that medications are taken, etc. Try to keep interventions to a minimum. With the client's consent, visitors can be encouraged to get involved in the provision of care for the client, where appropriate, during the visit.

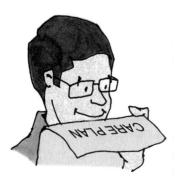

Take the opportunity, when required, to provide time and space for visitors to discuss their feelings, concerns, and needs in relation to the plan of care. Inform visitors about relevant support services and facilities that are available to them and where they can obtain further information.

Information provided or discussed with visitors should be consistent with the wishes of the client and the needs of the visitor(s). Adhere to any restrictions on movement by the client or visitor and levels of supervision, and ensure the level of privacy that is required throughout the visit (e.g., making sure that the client and visitor are not accidentally disturbed by others).

Ensure that any disputes between the client and others do not escalate to violence. This may necessitate

you in ending the visit prematurely. Assess the quality of interaction and enjoyment experienced by the client during the visit.

Exercise 3.9 🖉

After a visit, check with the client and visitors on the success of the visit (e.g., level of privacy, amount of time available, the maintenance of a positive relationship during the visit). Make a record and inform an appropriate member of the care team when visitors want to discuss issues which are outside your responsibilities, when they are experiencing problems in supporting the client during a visit, and/or when significant others appear to have a detrimental effect on the health or welfare of the client.

Prepare a short report on the success of the visit for inclusion within the client's records. Complete the necessary documentation required by any incident that has occurred during the visit (e.g., the client falling and injuring him/herself, complaints made by visitors).

If required, enable the client to change clothes on return from a visit. Also, ensure that any valuables given to the client are safely stored away, according to the client's wishes.

Exercise 3.10 🖉

Enabling Carers to Support Clients

The term "carer" in this situation includes friends and relatives of the client, individuals who provide regular or part-time care within the client's home (e.g., a neighbour), and those who provide care in a residential setting, but are not employed by the home (e.g., a volunteer).

The aim of supporting others is to help them become as independent as possible. Therefore, be careful that you do not allow anyone to become unnecessarily dependent on you. It is best if you can agree the type and amount of support that the carer requires so that he or she, in turn, can support the client.

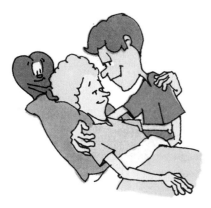

Help the carers to support their loved ones. Ensure that the support is provided in a manner which is most likely to make the carer and the client feel valued and respected whilst sustaining their relationship.

There are many areas in which a carer may need help when supporting a client (e.g., the provision of health care; help with managing finances or finding out about and accessing available services and facilities; general advice, support, and counselling to enable the carer to cope).

It is important that you are clear about your role in providing support to carers in terms of the limits of your responsibility and the limits of your competence. When you are unsure how to support a client or you are asked to provide a support service that is not within your usual work role, contact your manager or an experienced colleague for advice.

Exercise 3.11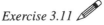

Where appropriate, provide information to the carer in a manner, and at a level and pace that allows clarification to be sought and questions answered (e.g., information on any potential difficulties that the carer may encounter with the client, the type and amount of help that is available, especially when a crisis occurs). This ensures that the information is fully understood and enables the client and carer to make informed decisions.

The type and level of support that is offered to a carer should reflect the needs and preferences of the client. For example, this may include accessing relief agencies, respite care, self-help groups, etc. The level

of support required by the carer and client is agreed with them and recorded in the client's record to ensure that all the care team are aware of the support that has been agreed.

If you suspect that there has been failure to care (e.g., signs of possible abuse, apparent neglect, or persistent and preventable problems keep occurring), contact the person-in-charge immediately. Appropriate steps need to be undertaken to improve the care that is being provided to the client without delay. See Module 1 for details about abuse.

When a client is (potentially) faced with moving to another care environment, your support should focus on assisting the client and carer to understand why the move is necessary. Also, you may be required to provide advice so that they can choose an appropriate care environment for the client (e.g., nursing home, residential care home, care at home or in a sheltered environment).

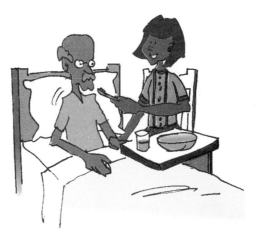

Sometimes a client and carer should be encouraged to undertake their own health care activities. Many health care activities are relatively simple and do not need to be carried out by a qualified health care professional.

The need for continuing care can be quite depressing, and the ability to be independent in the provision of health care can be a real morale booster. It allows the client and carer to fit the health care activities within the "normal flow" of the day, rather than be dependent on others.

The care worker's role is to provide the necessary support and encouragement so that the health care activities are completed according to the agreed plan of care. The aim is that the client receives a quality of care that is as good as that provided by qualified and experienced health care workers.

When a carer is expected to care for a client, this can change the relationship between them (e.g., the carer resents the change to his or her lifestyle; the carer feels there is no choice but to provide care for the client; the carer feels unsupported and helpless). Be aware that carers can feel very vulnerable and experience both physical and emotional stress when supporting clients.

Stress is evident when a carer admits to finding it very difficult to cope or shows signs of being unable to cope (e.g., becoming easily irritated, making mistakes that he or she would not normally make). The carer may show physical and mental signs of stress (e.g., appearing depressed, finding it difficult to think clearly, suffering from a number of minor illnesses such as stomach upsets, backache).

Exercise 3.12 🖎

The following are examples of procedures, treatments, and dressings that a client or carer may want to take on:

- **Dressings** (e.g., to wounds, pressure sores, leg ulcers)
- **Care of lesions** (e.g., skin treatments for psoriasis and eczema)
- **Elimination** (e.g., catheter care, changing urine drainage bags, prevention and management of constipation, stoma care, continence management)
- **Pressure area** care
- **Manual handling** (the carer learning how to move a client or the client learning how to move him/herself)
- Managing **challenging behaviour**

- **Infection control** (e.g., if a member of the family is HIV positive)
- Management of **epileptic seizures**
- **Tube feeding** for clients who cannot eat or drink orally
- **Personal hygiene** (e.g., bed baths, use of special bathing equipment)
- **Self-medication** of a variety of drugs

The following are examples of physical measurements and specimen collections that a client or carer may want to take on:

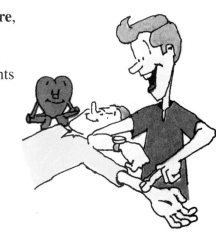

- **Temperature, pulse**, and **respiration** measurements
- **Blood pressure** measurements
- **Weight, height**, and **girth** measurements
- **Peak flow** measurements
- **Fluid balance** measurements
- **Blood** specimen collection and analysis
- **Urine** specimen collection and analysis
- **Faeces, sputum**, and **exudate** specimen collection

Exercise 3.13 🖎

Ensure that the carer and client are happy to undertake the health care activity. Encourage and support the carer to develop the necessary skills for the client's care, according to the agreed plan of care. You may be required to demonstrate or teach the carer the necessary care skill. Encourage the client or carer to be as independent as possible, although total independence in undertaking health care activities may never be achieved.

When the agreed plan of care highlights the need to maintain records, the carer or client should be encouraged/assisted to complete the necessary documentation. Records must be accurate, legible, complete, and stored in a safe place.

Some individuals may wish to use home remedies in conjunction with the treatments that have been prescribed. Encourage them to seek advice from the doctor. Home remedies may affect the action of the prescribed treatment.

Where available, provide leaflets and information packs to the client and carer on specific clinical procedures and health care problems, relevant services and facilities (e.g., medical waste collection). Provide contact numbers of relevant voluntary organisations that are concerned with the client's health problems.

If you have reason to suspect that standards of care are not being maintained, the carer should be encouraged and supported to discuss the problem and identify potential solutions. Do not be afraid to involve other members of the care team in this process, especially when you are asked questions that you cannot answer.

Exercise 3.14

Part 2: Supporting Others When Their Care Changes (W3)

Help clients to adapt to changes in their care.

The most common reason to change a person's care environment is because the required care service (e.g., cancer care) may only be available from another care agency or at a different location. This usually happens because the client's care needs have changed and cannot be met in the current care environment (e.g., a client in a residential home has to be transferred to a nursing home as care needs increase; a client, whose self-care abilities improve, is transferred to independent accommodation). For some clients, the transfer occurs on a regular basis (e.g., a client who is admitted to a residential care home for respite care once a month to give the carer a break). Also, when a client recovers from an illness in hospital, he or she is usually discharged home or transferred to a community care facility to recuperate.

Sometimes the change of care environment is unavoidable because of planned changes within the care organisation. A care facility may transfer to another (part of the) building/organisation, the facility may be closing or changing the type of care that is provided within that care environment.

In some instances, the client's age will necessitate transfer to an adult or elderly care facility. Occasionally, the bed or place that the client is occupying at the facility is required by someone who is more in need of that type of care (e.g., a client is transferred from an intensive care unit to a medical ward as his condition improves). In the private sector, the client may no longer be able to afford to stay at the chosen care facility.

Exercise 3.15

The value based requirements of good practice are particularly important within this area of care:

- Anti-discriminatory practice is actively promoted.

- The confidentiality of information is maintained to meet statutory and agency requirements.

- Individual rights and choice are actively promoted and supported.

- Personal beliefs and preferences are appropriately acknowledged.

- Individuals are supported by the use of effective communication.

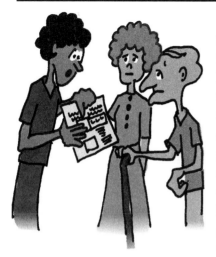

Whatever the reason(s) for the transfer, these may have to be explained to the client, family, and friends. Provide appropriate information about the care environment to which the client is being transferred. (This can be given verbally; leaflets, brochures, and maps may be available.) Answer their questions concerning the transfer in an acceptable manner and at a level and pace that enables them to understand what you are saying. Where possible, a client should be given the opportunity to indicate the person he or she would prefer to be the key contact and to identify care workers to contact in relation to the transfer.

Exercise 3.16

If, for any reason, the client and/or family and friends do not understand you, you will have to communicate your information to them in a different way (e.g., interpreter, Makaton signer). Refer them to a more experienced colleague if you cannot answer their questions or cannot make them understand.

If an unconscious client is being transferred, remember that the sense of hearing is the last sense to go and the first to return. Therefore, the transfer will need to be explained to the client at all stages.

Some clients will not want to move. Try to help them overcome their fears and anxieties by acknowledging their doubts and by carefully and sensitively explaining the reasons for the transfer. Do not be surprised if a planned transfer causes heightened emotional states (e.g., anxiety, anger) in individuals, especially if they disagree with and/or are apprehensive about the move. Help people cope with their strong feelings, and ensure that they do not adversely affect the plan of care.

You may experience some sympathy with the client and the family when they do not agree with the transfer decision. This is especially likely if the reason for the move is to meet the needs of the organisation (e.g., the facility is closing), or if you are not sure that the transfer will be in the client's best interests (e.g., the client is being discharged home early so that another client can be admitted for care).

Exercises 3.17 and 3.18

Preparing for the Transfer

A transfer to a new care environment often requires a great deal of thought and planning. Whenever possible, the client should make his or her own arrangements for the transfer. Make arrangements for transport or an escort, as needed. Make sure that the correct client is being transferred (e.g., from surgical ward to operating theatre). With the client's consent, inform relevant people about the transfer (e.g., significant others, care professionals).

If possible, prepare the new care environment for the client's arrival (e.g., transferring the client's possessions, ensuring that necessary medications and medical equipment are available for transfer with the client). Inform the client, family, and friends, and all necessary authorities if any legal or local policy conditions are attached to the transfer (e.g., a place of safety order for a child, a client sectioned under the Mental Health Act, access restriction such as visiting hours). Prepare the necessary transfer records. These should be accurate, legible, and neat so that they can be passed on to the person-in-charge of the client's new care environment or to the client's GP if he or she is being transferred home.

Exercise 3.19

During the transfer, the aim is to make the transition from one care environment to another as smooth and trouble-free as possible. Make sure that the client is comfortable and, if necessary, physically supported during the transfer. Administer medications and provide care, as required by the plan of care. If the client and others are kept waiting, explain the reasons for the delay, and keep them informed of developments whilst making them comfortable (e.g., providing meals, tea).

Observe the behaviour and condition of the client who is being transferred and any others who are accompanying the client. If there is cause for concern, take appropriate action (e.g., speed up the transfer, return to the original care environment, make a call for help). Be prepared to answer questions (e.g., How long will it take to get there? Will the escort/relative be able to stay for a while until the client settles in?).

After the transfer, anxiety and forgetfulness can result in the initial introductions to a new care environment having to be modified and/or repeated. Also, some clients can become totally disoriented and confused in a new care environment, even when they have previously been mentally alert and the transfer has been carefully and repeatedly explained to them.

If the client becomes confused or disoriented on transfer, orient the client to the new care environment whilst maintaining the client's safety within the plan of care. Some clients can take a long time to adjust to a new care environment, especially if they find it difficult to cope with change. In addition, if the client is blind, he or she will have to get used to the layout of the new environment and the positioning of possessions.

First impressions count. Provide a friendly welcome, and explain information about the new care environment in a way that is easily understood by the client and significant others. You may have to describe any new forms of care that are to be provided, including any aspects of care that are likely to cause distress to the client (e.g., locked doors, having to share a bedroom). Explain how to summon help.

Provide a tour of the new care environment. If available, provide the client with a plan of the layout or draw a diagram. Explain any restrictions or rights of access (e.g., visiting times, secure accommodation).

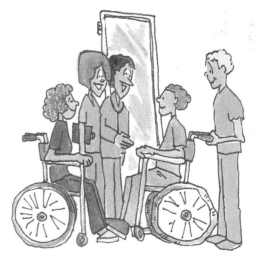

Introduce relevant others (e.g., care staff, other clients), and explain what facilities are available. Ask whether there are any arrangements that will be needed to help the client adapt to the new environment (e.g., arranging the client's personal belongings, ensuring that the care workers are aware of the client's preferences in terms of nourishment, times for going to bed).

It is essential that the client's adjustment to the new environment is monitored and any relevant actions are taken that can help the client to adjust to the new environment (e.g., frequent visits from relatives, bringing in personal belongings). If specified in the plan of care, record the client's progress in adjusting to the new care environment.

Exercise 3.20

Summary

Promote clients' interests, identity, and emotional well-being by encouraging and supporting them in leisure pursuits and keeping in contact with their significant others. Help them to plan and undertake visits and to receive visitors. Whenever possible, family and friends should be encouraged and supported to provide care for the clients.

Transferring clients to new care environments often requires a great deal of thought and planning. Clients especially need your support when undergoing a change in the provision of care if it is to be successful.

Check Your Knowledge and Understanding

1. You are caring for a client who has a broken forearm which has been placed in a plaster cast. He is frustrated at not being able to play rugby, and he is frightened that he will lose his high levels of fitness during his enforced lay off. Which of the following would you do?

   a) Reassure him by highlighting that, because he is so fit at the moment, he will soon regain his fitness when he resumes playing rugby again.

   b) Suggest that he concentrates on more sedentary hobbies and pastimes until his arm has healed.

   c) Suggest that he get some advice from the physiotherapist on how to ensure that his arm is properly protected and supported whilst continuing general fitness training, until he can resume the contact sport of rugby.

   d) Suggest that he continue his rugby training, but avoids playing rugby until he has been given the all-clear by his doctor.

2. A client who enjoys train spotting goes to the local station, noting the numbers of trains, spending a lot of time and energy on this activity. Recently, you have received a complaint from the station master outlining how the client is "bothering" the train drivers by attempting to have conversations with them. How should this situation be handled?

   a) Ignore the letter because the client has a right to talk to the train drivers if he so chooses.

   b) Contact the station master at the earliest opportunity to find out what the client is doing that has led to him writing this letter. Then negotiate with the station master a plan of action to overcome this "problem" whilst ensuring that the client can continue his train-spotting hobby.

   c) Write a letter of complaint to the station master outlining how your client's rights are being infringed by his outmoded attitude.

   d) Contact the station master at the earliest opportunity to find out what the client is doing that has led to him writing this letter. Share this information with the client, and get his views on the situation. If necessary, observe the client's behaviour at the station. Then decide what to do about the "problem."

3. It has been arranged for one of your clients, a young man who has previously been abused by one of his parents, to go to a local football match for the first time with his brother. When the brother arrives to pick up him up, he is very scruffy, has "love" and "hate" tattooed on his knuckles, and has a lot of facial piercing to his ears, nose, lips, and tongue. The old and rusty car in which he arrived contains two other young men who are similar in appearance.

   When you engage the man in conversation, he promises to look after his brother and return him by six o'clock that evening. Whilst you are talking to the man, his two friends in the car are shouting football slogans and singing football songs to passers-by. The brother turns round to his two friends and shouts "Shut your gobs, you w***ers!" The appearance and attitude of the three young men who are accompanying the client to the football match, worry you. What should you do?

a)   Simply accept that the man will look after his brother and return him safely, as previously arranged.

b)   Ask the brother and his friends to promise to tone down their language whilst your client is in their company.

c)   Refuse to allow your client to be taken out by these "undesirables."

d)   Immediately call a meeting of the care staff who are on duty to discuss whether it is desirable for your client to go to the football match with his brother.

4.   One of your clients has decided that he would like to write to his sister who lives 200 miles away. When he has finished the letter, he hands it to you, together with an envelope and a postage stamp, and asks you to post it to his sister. The letter is written in green crayon on a large scrap of paper. There are lots of spelling errors, and it is very scruffy. What should you do?

a)   Simply put the letter in the envelope and seal it, add the address and postage stamp, and then post it to his sister.

b)   Ask the client if you can neatly rewrite the letter so that his sister can read it more easily, and then post it to his sister.

c)   Inform the client that he should address his own envelope, put the letter inside, and stick on the stamp before you will post it for him.

d)   Rewrite the letter, without telling the client, and then post it to his sister.

5.   You have gone into town accompanied by two clients from a children's home where you work. You are returning to the home when you meet up with one of the children's previous foster parents. This child is on the "at risk" register because it has been suspected (but not proven) that the child has been sexually abused by these foster parents. The couple insist that they should be allowed to take the child home to play for the afternoon, although the child's plan of care states that they should be supervised at all times when with the child. What would you do?

a)   Tell the couple that you suspect that they have previously sexually abused the child and that an unsupervised home visit is out of the question.

b)   Inform the couple that the care plan states that the couple must be supervised at all times when with the child. Therefore, they are not allowed to take the child home.

c)   Same as "b," except that you inform the couple that, if they write to the manager of the home, it should be possible to organise a member of staff to accompany the child and provide supervision during a future visit to their house.

d)   Allow the couple to take the child home for a couple of hours, as long as they promise to look after her properly.

6.   You are caring for a client who has been having treatment for an AIDS-related health problem. He has informed the care team that he does not want anyone to know his diagnosis. His family approach you one day and insist that their son's diagnosis and treatment should be clearly explained to them. They say they are not willing to be fobbed off with explanations such as "he has a chest problem." What would you do?

a)   Inform them that the client has requested that his diagnosis and treatment remain confidential.

b)   Inform them that they must ask the client if they want further information.

c) Inform them of the diagnosis as they have a right to know, but request that they do not embarrass the client by letting him know that they know.

d) Refer the relatives to the person-in-charge.

7. You have an elderly relative who has recently moved from a residential care home to a nursing home as he has become more dependent on others for his care. The nursing home staff have a set routine and have made it clear that they would prefer you not to provide care for your relative when you visit him. What would you do?

a) Comply with the wishes of the care staff, as long as your relative appears to be receiving good care.

b) Negotiate with the care team and the relative a plan of care that includes your input into the provision of care.

c) Make a formal complaint to the nursing home manager about the inappropriateness of an enforced routine and your exclusion from care involvement.

d) Immediately withdraw your relative from the home.

8. You are talking to an elderly and frail carer who looks after her disabled husband at home. She is having severe financial problems at the moment, struggling to cope on their joint pension and a small amount of savings. The house is cold, and you suspect that the couple have not been eating properly for a while. You suggest to her that they are probably eligible for welfare benefits, but the couple insist that they will never accept "charity." What would you do?

a) Accept that the couple will never claim welfare benefits.

b) Offer to review the couple's finances to see if there is a better way of managing their income.

c) Inform the carer that you will mention this situation to your supervisor, and ask them if they would be willing to talk through their financial problems with an appropriately qualified officer.

d) Insist that the carer visit the welfare benefit office so that she can get further advice on the subject.

Module 4

Contributing to Health, Safety, and Security

Provide an environment that is healthy, safe, and secure for everyone.

Need-to-know words:

- acidosis
- angina
- antibody
- audit
- CPR
- crepitus
- cross-infection
- defibrillation
- disinfection
- first aid
- fracture
- Heimlich manoeuvre
- hyperglycaemia
- hypoglycaemia
- ketones
- micro-organisms
- protective barriers
- seizure
- sharps
- sterilisation
- stroke
- tumour
- Universal Precautions

Objectives:

- Explain the principles of client security.
- Outline the management of cash and valuables.
- Explain how to prevent accidents.
- Discuss relevant legislation covering health and safety.
- Outline how to deal with environmental emergencies.
- Demonstrate safe manual handling.
- Utilise the principles of infection control.
- Demonstrate how to deal with health emergencies.

Module 4 Introduction

Module 4 relates to just one unit of the level 2 NVQ/SVQ Award in Care:

Unit CU1: **Promote, Monitor, and Maintain Health, Safety, and Security in the Workplace** is a mandatory group A unit that consists of three elements of competence:

- CU1.1   Monitor and maintain the safety and security of the work environment.

- CU1.2   Promote standards of health and safety in working practice.

- CU1.3   Minimise the risks arising from health emergencies.

Part 1:   Maintaining Health, Safety, and Security   (CU1)

Simple precautions prevent serious injuries and maintain security.

This unit covers a wide range of subject areas—safety and security, health and safety at work, lifting and moving, infection control, and first aid.

The **security** of the people in your care is very important and generally relates to three main issues—legal, clinical, and personal safety.

- *Legal reasons* (e.g., a child provided with a "place of safety," a person referred to a regional secure unit for assessment)

- *Clinical reasons* (e.g., a person who needs regular medication or treatment, a person with an infection who is isolated)

- *Personal safety reasons* (e.g., a person with a learning disability who might wander off and suffer from exposure, a person who may attempt to take his or her own life)

Establishments have different levels and methods of security. For example, a special hospital might lock all client rooms at night; use cameras, alarms and special lighting; or employ security staff to monitor entrances and exits. In contrast, a psychiatric hospital might only lock up a small area (such as a secure ward) and make regular checks for the presence of clients.

Exercise 4.1 🖉

Whatever the level of security of the building, you need to be sure of your legal rights to prevent someone from leaving or entering. Establish rights of entry before allowing callers to enter the premises. If you have an appointments system, stick to it unless there is good reason for not doing so. Carefully explain any restrictions on a person's freedom to the person involved, and ensure that all staff know about the restrictions. If a client who cannot be prevented from leaving is likely to wander off and be in danger, clearly state in the care plan the level and type of supervision for this person.

Missing Client

If a person goes missing, search the building thoroughly. Then search the grounds and local areas. Ask the staff and other clients to see if anyone knows where the person might have gone. If not found, the person-in-charge will have to set in motion the missing person procedure. This includes making a note of when the person was last seen, when it was noticed that the person was missing, what the person was wearing when last seen, and if there are any restrictions on freedom.

Police need to be contacted, especially, if the person is legally not allowed to leave the building or if the person is likely to be in any danger. The police will want the same details listed previously, plus they will want a description of the person. They will also want to know about any places or people that the missing person is likely to visit and whether the person is dangerous.

Ensure that all details concerning this incident are clearly written up in the person's care plan and on any forms that are required.

Exercise 4.2 🖉

Keeping Money and Valuables Safe

Encourage people to keep their personal belongings in secure and appropriate places. Discourage vulnerable people from keeping too much money or too many valuables on them. Ensure that you know and follow any policies or procedures for handling money and valuables.

Lock the expensive equipment away when not in use. Keep the equipment inventory up-to-date so that it is easy to check if something goes missing. Mark all expensive equipment by engraving and/or writing a security code in ultra violet-sensitive ink. Secure buildings during the day and night as appropriate.

If valuables go missing or are stolen, the police will almost certainly be called in, and everybody will be under suspicion. Anyone found guilty of stealing will probably be dismissed. If you have any concerns regarding health, safety, and security, seek advice from an appropriate person (e.g., health and safety officer, security officer, fire officer, the police).

Exercise 4.3 🖉

Ensuring Safe Environments

The Health and Safety at Work Act (1974) identifies responsibilities for the employer, the employee, and the management for ensuring a safe environment.

Employee duties include caring for the health and safety of self and others, and complying with the requirements imposed on the employer. Adhere to instructions in the operation of the plant and equipment,

and use materials only according to recommended procedures. Use protective clothing and equipment, as directed. Never interfere or misuse anything provided for health, safety, and welfare.

Employer duties include ensuring the health, safety, and welfare at work for all employees, and providing and maintaining equipment and systems that are safe. Employers also provide information, instruction, training, and supervision for health and safety at work.

Management responsibilities include maintaining a safe environment for all staff; ensuring that staff adhere to health and safety orders, policies, and procedures; and providing training for safe practices and work methods. Management duties also include explaining hazards and safe practices to new employees before they commence work. They also are responsible for the recording all accidents.

Maintain an environment of health, safety, and security based on allowing people who are receiving care to have individual choice in furnishings, activities, etc., that are consistent with organisational policies. Take appropriate action immediately whenever a person's health, safety, or security is threatened.

Record all accidents and incidents carefully and comprehensively in accordance with local and national policies, and keep your manager informed of events. If you have any concerns about health, safety, or security, seek advice from an appropriate person (e.g., your local health and safety representative).

Be a good role model for others. Dress, behave, and practice personal hygiene in keeping with good health and safety practices, including the use of appropriate protection where necessary.

Exercise 4.4 🖉

55

Control of Substances Hazardous to Health (COSHH) regulations require employers to assess the risks created at work where hazardous substances are used. Facts that must be identified include potential risks from using the substance in the place of work, how the risks are to be managed, and what precautions should be taken in terms of storage, usage, disposal, etc. The employer must provide training for all aspects of working with dangerous substances.

Consider simple strategies for your personal safety, especially in the community.

- Carefully preview the day's cases to check whether anybody who is in your care is potentially violent.
- Ask to have a colleague present, take an escort, or use a taxi, if unsure.
- Leave your itinerary and expected departure/ arrival times.
- Tell colleagues, manager, etc., about possible changes to the plan.
- Arrange for contact if your return is overdue.
- Carry a personal alarm or portable telephone.
- Refrain from carrying a bag/briefcase, or wearing an outer uniform, or having car stickers that suggest you have money or drugs with you.
- Make sure you have an out-of-hours telephone number to summon help if needed.

Exercise 4.5 ✏

Preventing Accidents

The best way to avoid an accident is to be alert to potential hazards by assessing the risk in any given situation. You have a duty to yourself, your family, your clients, and your colleagues to remain vigilant. If you notice a potential hazard, you may need to follow one or more of these general guidelines:

- Get out of harm's way.
- Remove, or make safe, the hazard, if possible.
- Label the hazard (e.g., "wet floors" sign).

- Inform an appropriate authority so that the hazard can be removed, replaced, or fixed.
- If appropriate, stay near the hazard so that you can keep others away.
- Inform everybody of the hazard at the earliest possibility.

Exercise 4.6 ✏

Falls are a significant cause of injury. The risk of falling is high for older people, usually due to general weakness, paralysis, confusion, dizziness, impaired vision, or other physical problems. Before making any changes to a person's immediate environment, ask the person for permission. This is a courtesy, as well as a safety factor.

Be alert to safety hazards, and take extra precautions to protect elderly and frail people from injury. Simple precautions can prevent serious injuries.

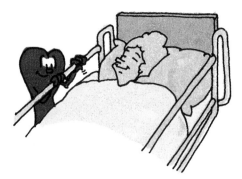

- Keep side rails up when the bed is occupied by someone who may fall out.
- Remove obstacles to walking such as personal belongings, wires, or equipment.
- Wipe up spills immediately, taking into consideration the substance that has been spilled and the appropriate safe method for disposal.
- Assist people in and out of the bath as appropriate.
- Use good lighting.
- Use good wheelchair technique. Lock wheels when moving people to and from wheelchairs, and ensure that feet are securely placed on the footrests when moving the wheelchair.

- Keep items that are used frequently close at hand so that the person does not fall reaching for them.

- Answer the call light promptly so that the person does not try to get up unaided. Do not leave helpless people unattended.

- Encourage people who are unsteady to use handrails and other prescribed mobility aids when walking.

- Assist with walking if needed.

- Be alert to furniture or objects that pose a hazard.

Burns and scalds are preventable. Enforce non-smoking policies to prevent fires and cigarette burns. Make sure that clients' bath water is not too hot. Test the water temperature yourself, and let the person who is having the bath test the water. Where appropriate, assist people with hot foods and liquids.

Exercise 4.7

Accidental poisoning can be the result of carelessness, confusion, or not being able to read labels because of poor vision. Keep all cleaning agents and disinfectants locked in appropriate storage cupboards. Never place them in household food containers; they may be mistaken for food.

Choking can be prevented by ensuring clients are positioned properly for eating and swallowing. Supervise clients carefully at meal times if they are at risk of choking, and encourage clients to take smaller bites and to eat more slowly.

Prevent **electrocution** by inspecting all electrical equipment externally for obvious damage (e.g., frayed wires). Ensure that all electrical equipment that is brought into the care facility is checked by an electrician. Operate all equipment according to instructions. If in doubt, ask.

Always ensure, where possible, that electrical equipment is properly earthed, and ensure that people and environments are dry before plugging in

equipment. Do not overload electrical circuits by using adaptors inappropriately, and avoid using extension leads whenever possible.

Exercise 4.8

Promoting Fire Safety

Fire can cause panic to fit and healthy people. For people confined to wheelchairs or beds, or who have reduced mobility, a fire can be terrifying. These people will be depending on you for their safety.

Awareness of fire hazards is the first step toward prevention. Three elements are needed for a fire to start; by removing any of the following elements, a fire can be prevented or put out:

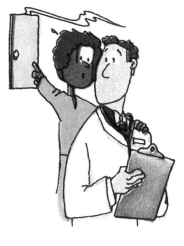

- **Heat:** Flame, spark, or other heat source
- **Oxygen:** Found in the air you breathe
- **Fuel:** Any combustible material (items that can catch fire and burn easily)

Alert the person-in-charge if you smell smoke. If a door feels hot, **do not open the door!**

Fire Hazards

Smoking: Never leave smokers unsupervised. Some people cannot handle smoking materials safely by themselves (due to medication, confusion, etc.). Smoking materials (e.g., cigarettes, pipes, tobacco, matches) should be safely stored when not being used. Strictly enforce the smoking policy, and allow smoking in authorised areas only. Never permit smoking near oxygen that is in use.

Be careful when you empty ashtrays, so that you do not set the rubbish bin on fire. Ensure the ashtrays are non-combustible, and never allow paper cups or rubbish bins to be used as ashtrays.

Exercise 4.9 🖉

Storage: Never store oily rags, paint cans, chemicals, or other combustibles in closed areas.

Electrical equipment: Inspect all electrical equipment that you use, and report any defects. Do not use faulty or potentially dangerous equipment (e.g., frayed electrical cables, overloaded circuits, overheated equipment, improperly earthed equipment).

Aerosol cans: The containers are likely to explode when they are exposed to heat. Never burn aerosol cans, never use an aerosol spray near open flames or cigarettes, and do not dispose of aerosol cans in rubbish bags that are to be incinerated.

In Case of Fire

Ensure that you know your organisation's emergency fire procedures.

- Understand fire evacuation procedures and designated assembly points where people can be counted to see if anyone is missing.
- Know locations of all exits and fire doors.
- Know where fire alarms and extinguishers are located.
- Know emergency telephone numbers.

In case of fire, remember: ARCE!

Alarm

   Rescue/evacuate

      Contain

         Extinguish

---

1. Sound the **alarm**.

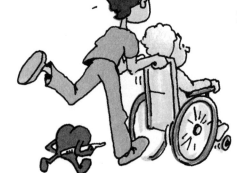

2. **Rescue** any people in immediate danger if it is safe to do so, and evacuate the premises.

3. **Contain** the fire by closing doors and windows.

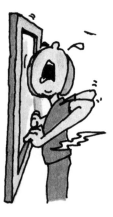

4. **Extinguish** the fire, if possible, using the correct extinguisher.

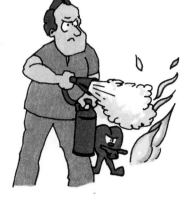

Exercise 4.10 🖉

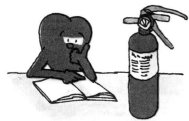

Fire Extinguishers

Different types of extinguishers are used for different types of fires. Be sure you have the correct extinguisher for the fire, or you may make the fire worse and put yourself in danger.

Water: (red) For most fires, except those involving flammable liquids or live electrical equipment

Foam: (cream/yellow) For burning liquids or electrical fires

Powder: (blue) For burning liquids or electrical fires

CO^2 Gas: (black) For burning liquids or electrical fires

Halon: (green) For electrical fires

AFFF: (cream/yellow) For general or electrical fires, or burning liquids. Use as directed for water or foam, depending on type of fire.

In addition, there should be a fire blanket in the kitchen. The fire blanket can be thrown over the blaze (e.g., chip pan fire) to smother the fire and minimise fire damage.

Exercise 4.11

Gas Escapes

Whenever you can smell gas or you suspect that there is a gas leak, open all windows and doors to let in as much fresh air as possible. Avoid anything that might cause the gas to explode (e.g., light a cigarette, put a light switch on, turn the central heating on or off). Ensure the gas board are called on their emergency telephone number to alert them as quickly as possible to deal with the gas leak.

Bomb Scares

If you receive a warning that a bomb has been planted somewhere in the building, you must immediately inform the person-in-charge. He or she should ensure that immediate evacuation of the building takes place, everyone congregates at the specified assembly points so that they can be checked and counted, and police are informed of the situation.

Part 2: Maintaining Personal Health and Safety (CU1.2)

Never take risks with your health at work.

You have a responsibility to yourself, your family, your colleagues, and your employer to ensure that you do not take chances with your health at work.

Safe Lifting and Moving

The Manual Handling Operations Regulations came into force in the United Kingdom in 1993. The regulations provide clear guidelines on moving and lifting practice for employers and employees as well as a framework for risk assessment. Each care organisation will have interpreted these regulations

in determining their own manual handling policies and procedures. Use only lifting and moving techniques that are sanctioned by your employing organisation.

The regulations have placed an emphasis away from the old philosophy of "safe lifting" to a philosophy of avoiding manual lifting whenever possible. The approach to lifting and moving should focus on adapting the task to suit the skills and physical abilities of those undertaking it. The expectation is that unavoidable handling tasks must be assessed in advance and action taken to remove or reduce the risk of injury to participants. Factors that should be taken into account during a risk assessment are the *task*, the *load* (e.g., shape, size, weight, and stability), the *environment*, and the individual *capabilities* of the staff.

It is expected that this process should be documented. If the task is deemed hazardous, mechanical lifting and handling aids should be made available. A lack of funds or resources is not an acceptable excuse for not providing the necessary training and equipment for manual handling.

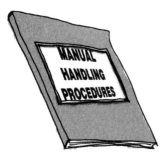

Lifting and moving is a major cause of accidents for care workers. A good employer will ensure that all care staff have access to a comprehensive education programme that includes the moving and handling of patients, minimising the risks, and utilising the best equipment available. Updates on manual handling should be provided annually.

Exercise 4.12

If you have not completed a manual handling course covering relevant techniques and mechanical aids to lifting and moving, you should not become involved in the manual handling of clients. If you have received appropriate training, protect yourself and others from injury by using only the approved manual handling techniques and equipment. Avoid any manual handling of clients unless the necessary resources are available, except in emergencies. If you have concerns about the moving and manual handling techniques used in your area of work, contact your manager, your organisation's manual handling coordinator (if there is one), your local health and safety officer, or your occupational health officer.

The problem is more difficult when a client refuses to be moved using manual handling aids. Fortunately, a client does not have the right to cause injury to a care worker by refusing the use of necessary equipment. If you encounter a problem in this area, seek advice from your manager.

Basic Handling Principles

Respect clients' wishes, whenever possible, when moving them or changing their positions. Maximise respect and dignity, and minimise any pain, discomfort, or friction during the move.

First, take a few seconds to assess the task at hand. Make sure that there is enough space to undertake the task, and prepare the environment for the move. If you need to change the environment to carry out the movement, ask the client's permission first. Then return the environment to its original state before you leave.

Ensure that everybody involved in the task has received appropriate, recent training. Check the clothing and footwear worn by all participants to make sure that there is no hindrance to movement.

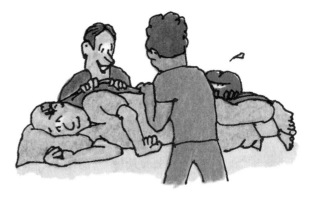

Tell the client what you are going to do, and encourage him or her to help and to be as mobile as possible. Ensure that privacy is maintained, where appropriate.

One carer can lift up to 25 kg (3 st 13 lb for men), 16.6 kg (2 st 8 lb for women), and no more. This applies only to loads held close to the lower body. Ensure that your spine does not twist during the task, and hold the load close to your body. If two (or more) carers are involved in the move, one should take the lead to coordinate all actions.

After the move, position the client safely and comfortably. Wash your hands before and after moving or positioning someone.

Do not use the drag lift to move clients. This is where the carers' arms are hooked under the clients' arms in order to drag that person (e.g., up a bed). Do not lift or move a client if the necessary equipment is not available. When in doubt, contact your organisation's manual handling coordinator or your manager for advice. For further information on the moving of clients, see Module 5.

Exercise 4.13

Infection Control

Infection control is critical! By understanding how infection spreads, you can protect yourself and others. Therefore, if you have an infection, it may not be appropriate for you to work. If there are no clear guidelines, ask your manager. Notify your manager immediately if you are ill with a notifiable disease (e.g., measles).

Infection is spread by micro-organisms (e.g., bacteria, viruses) that can only be seen with a microscope. Micro-organisms are everywhere—in the air, on your skin, in food and beverages, and in everything that you touch. There are two types of organisms—*non-pathogenic* (harmless), and *pathogenic* (harmful).

Pathogens are spread in three ways:

- **Through the air**, via people coughing and sneezing (e.g., common cold, diptheria)

- **By direct contact** with another person, by touching contaminated objects, from animals and insects, by ingesting contaminated food or water (e.g., salmonella food poisoning), sexually transmitted diseases, or glandular fever from kissing

- **Through blood and blood products** via an injection or inoculation through broken skin (e.g., rabies, hepatitis B virus)

Micro-organisms that cause disease include *bacteria* (e.g., mycobacterium tuberculosis causes **TB**), *viruses* (e.g., human immunodeficiency virus **causes AIDS**), and *fungi* (e.g., candida albicans causes thrush).

Infection usually enters the body through broken or damaged skin, or through the mucous membranes of the eyes, nose, air passages, and digestive tract. Always report the following potential signs of infection:

- Fever
- Chills
- Restlessness
- Swelling
- Redness
- Pain
- Lack of appetite
- Behaviour changes
- Discharge

Exercise 4.14

Minimise the spread of infection through keeping the environment clean and tidy, sterilisation and disinfection, good linen handling, and isolation.

Sterilisation kills all micro-organisms that are on an object. Unless they are all dead, the object is not sterile. A sterile object becomes contaminated when exposed to air or when touched by non-sterile objects. Surgical equipment is always sterilised after use. It is either *autoclaved* (an intense heat process) or *cold sterilised* by soaking the object in an approved disinfectant for a set length of time.

Disinfection uses chemical (disinfectants) to kill most micro-organisms. Those that are not killed have their growth slowed. Examples here are disinfectant sprays for work surfaces and equipment that are **sanitised**—washed in disinfectant, dried, and stored.

Exercise 4.15

Linen Handling

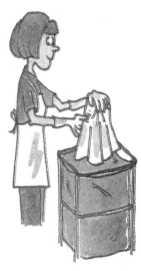

Use precautions whenever you handle linen to prevent infection from spreading. Hold linen away from you to avoid transferring micro-organisms. Avoid shaking or fluffing linen, and keep the linen off the floor.

Wear gloves to handle linen that is soiled with excrement, blood, or body fluids. Place soiled linen in covered hampers or bags to prevent the spread of infection and to control odours. Always wash your hands after handling soiled linen.

Isolation

Isolation (setting apart) procedures are used when extra precautions are necessary to control the spread of infection. People with contagious diseases are sometimes isolated to protect others from becoming infected. Isolation may also be ordered for people who cannot fight infection because of age, illness, or treatment. Doctors prescribe isolation precautions which vary according to the specific problem. It is very important to follow isolation procedures.

Signs are posted on the door requiring visitors to report to the person-in-charge before entering. Surgical gowns, gloves, and masks may be required, depending on the type of infection.

All basic supplies and equipment for the care of an isolated person should be stored in the person's room. Gather any additional equipment before you put on a gown and enter the room.

It is not uncommon for an isolated person to become depressed. You can help prevent depression in a variety of ways:

- Answer the call light promptly.
- Care for the isolated person first.

- Tell the person when you will be back. Try to be prompt, and let the person know if you are going to be delayed.
- Be cautious of what you say outside the room as the person may hear you.
- Help the person, the person's family, and any other visitors to be comfortable and confident with isolation procedures.
- Provide puzzles, books and other amusements to keep the person occupied.

Exercise 4.16 🖉

Washing Your Hands

Washing your hands regularly is the single most effective preventive measure for infection control. Most of the time you will wash your hands in soap and water, taking care to wash all aspects of the hands and fingers, and ensuring that the hands are thoroughly dried afterwards.

Before any clinical activity, wash your hands with bacteriocidal soap (rather than ordinary soap), or wash your hands with bacteriocidal alcohol hand rub.

Exercise 4.17 🖉

WASH YOUR HANDS

- Before and after work
- Before and after meals
- Before and after providing care
- After using the toilet
- After coughing, sneezing, or blowing your nose
- After handling bedpan specimens, body fluids, or human tissue
- After handling soiled linen

Protective Barriers

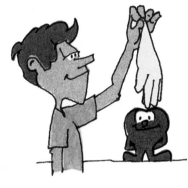

Protective equipment provides a barrier between you and the sources of infection. Appropriate equipment such as masks, gloves, and gowns should be worn whenever you could be exposed to infection. In addition, keep your own cuts and abrasions covered by a waterproof plaster or dressing.

Wear medical **gloves** when you have contact with any of the following:

- People who are bleeding or have open wounds
- Blood or other body fluids
- Soiled linen

When **putting on gloves**, check for cracks, punctures, tears or discolouration, and discard them if they are damaged. Check that they are a good fit. If a gown is worn, pull the gloves over the gown cuffs.

When **removing gloves**, take hold of the glove at the cuff and pull it inside out. Hold the removed glove in the hand that is still gloved. Then take hold of the second glove at the cuff, and pull that one inside out, enclosing the first glove in the second glove. Dispose of the gloves using the designated bin for infected waste, and wash your hands.

Exercise 4.18 🖉

Universal Precautions were developed to prevent the spread of deadly blood-borne viruses and bacteria. The precautions establish safe practices for care workers to control the spread of the human immunodeficiency virus (HIV) and the hepatitis B virus (HBV). Infected people often have no symptoms and may not know they are infected. Therefore, consider yourself at risk of infection from everyone.

Treat *everyone* with care, and use precaution for each person receiving care, all used needles, all body fluids, and body waste. Assume all are potentially infectious. Gloves must be worn at all times when handling these materials to avoid infection.

Blood, faeces, urine, sweat, vomit, and nose and mouth secretions are sources of cross-infection (infection passed from one person to another). Always wear gloves when handling these materials.

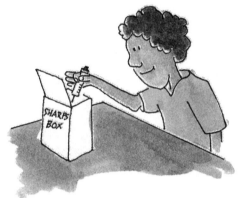

Everyone who handles **sharps** (e.g., needles) must use extra caution. You are personally responsible for the disposal of the sharps that you use. Be aware that gloves will not protect you from a needle stick injury (pricking yourself with a used needle). Never re-sheath needles. Dispose of sharps directly into a sharps bin. Never fill a sharps bin more than 3/4 full, and close the bin securely, before disposal. Where appropriate, get yourself vaccinated against hepatitis B.

Other precautions include the following:

- If you are pregnant and working in a high-risk area, seek advice from your manager.
- Report all broken skin, any contact with potentially infected materials, and all puncture wounds, according to your organisation's policies.
- Cover spills of blood with chlorine granules, and then mop up after two minutes.

- Discard excreta directly into the drainage system.
- Use yellow bags for contaminated waste.

Exercise 4.19 🖉

Clinical Waste

All individuals and organisations who produce clinical (controlled) waste have a duty of care in relation to its safe storage and disposal, according to the Environmental Protection Act (1990). Prevent others from illegally disposing of waste. Safely store and package waste so that it cannot escape whilst being stored or during transit for its disposal. Ensure that waste is only given to an authorised authority for disposal, and provide a written description of the waste.

It is recommended, unless there is a fully justified reason for not doing so, that all clinical waste should be incinerated. In addition, under the Control of Substances Hazardous to Health Regulations (1994), the risks of storing and disposing of clinical waste have to be assessed. This necessitates policies for the management of clinical waste including specification of containers that are to be used for clinical waste and measures for the safe storage, transport, and handling of waste. Staff training is necessary for all levels of staff who may come into contact with the waste, and personal protection must be available. Report all accidents.

If, for any reason, you become involved in the disposal of "special waste" (e.g., radioactive materials, cytotoxic drugs), contact the infection control officer at your nearest NHS Trust. The only exemptions to the duty of care in the management of clinical waste are for occupiers of domestic properties.

Exercise 4.20 🖉

Part 3: Responding to Health Emergencies (CU1.3)

Your prompt action can save lives.

Emergencies happen. Someone's life may depend on you, and you must act fast. Remember, though, that you can worsen the injuries of a casualty if you do not know what you are doing. The following sections provide an *overview* of basic first aid skills. You need to attend a first aid course to learn the practice of first aid.

Exercise 4.21 🖉

Principles of First Aid

First aid is emergency care for a person who is ill or injured, before medical help arrives. First aid is given to prevent death or to keep injuries from getting worse.

- Act quickly, giving priority to the most urgent conditions.

- Check that there is no further danger to the casualty or to yourself.
- Check the casualty for responsiveness by gently shaking the shoulders and asking, "Are you all right?"
- If the casualty responds, leave the person in the position in which you found him or her, as long as there is no danger.
- Reassess the casualty regularly, and position correctly.
- If the casualty does not respond, shout for help and check the airway.
- If breathing has stopped, clear the airway, and begin cardiopulmonary resuscitation.
- Control bleeding.
- Guard against shock.

- Give reassurance to the casualty and to onlookers.
- If you must move the casualty, immobilise fractures and dress large wounds.
- If needed, get the casualty to hospital for medical treatment as soon as possible.
- Observe carefully for any changes in the casualty's condition.
- Do not try to do too much yourself.
- Do not give anything by mouth to a casualty who is unconscious or who may need an anaesthetic on arrival at hospital.
- Always record emergency incidents accurately and comprehensively in the prescribed format.

Exercise 4.22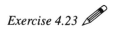

Signs and symptoms of the different emergency situations may differ with the casualty's age and ethnicity. For example, an old person may fracture a femur (thigh bone) during a very minor fall and not show the level of pain you would expect from a major leg fracture. Another example is difficulty in detecting bruising and pallor in people who have darker skins.

When someone requires first aid, other people tend to be drawn to the situation. Some may be concerned and would like to help; others will simply have a morbid fascination for watching. Health emergencies have an effect on anyone who is nearby, especially if they are friends or relatives. You may need to send someone to get help, ask onlookers to stand back to give the casualty air, to keep clear of any danger, and to give you plenty of room. Provide first aid to onlookers if they are shocked or faint, and ask for support when someone is feeling upset by the incident.

Recovery Position

The recovery position is used for casualties who have fainted or are unconscious. It is used to prevent the casualty from choking on the tongue or on vomit, especially if the person is unconscious and lying on the back.

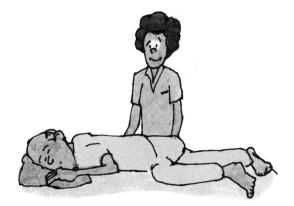

1. If necessary, remove the casualty's spectacles.
2. Kneel beside the casualty and make sure that the legs are straight.
3. Open the airway by tilting the head and lifting the chin.
4. Tuck the arm nearest to you well under the buttock on the same side, arm straight and palm uppermost.
5. Fetch the far arm across the chest, and hold the back of the hand against the casualty's nearest cheek.
6. With your other hand, grasp the far leg just above the knee and pull it up, keeping the foot on the ground.
7. Keeping the hand pressed against the cheek, pull on the leg to roll the victim toward you onto the side.
8. Adjust the upper leg so that both the hip and knee are bent at right angles.
9. Adjust the lower arm so that the casualty is not lying on it and the palm is still uppermost.
10. Tilt the head back to make sure the airway remains open.
11. Adjust the hand under the cheek if necessary, to keep the head tilted.
12. Check breathing.

Exercise 4.23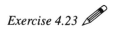

Shock

All casualties experience a certain amount of shock. It is important for you to recognise the signs and symptoms of shock.

- The casualty feels sick, vomits, or may be thirsty.
- The skin is pale, cold, clammy, and may be sweating.
- Breathing becomes shallow and rapid with yawning and sighing.
- Pulse rate becomes quicker, but weaker.
- Unconsciousness may develop.

The treatment for shock aims at getting an adequate supply of blood to the brain and vital organs. Follow these guidelines for treating shock:

- Reassure the casualty.

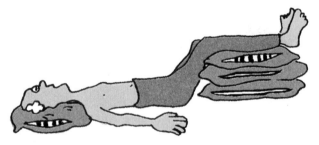

- Lay the casualty down, and raise the legs if possible.
- Place in the recovery position if the person becomes unconscious.
- Loosen tight clothing to help circulation and breathing.
- Moisten the lips if the casualty is thirsty (but do not give anything to drink).
- Avoid moving the casualty unnecessarily.
- Begin cardiopulmonary resuscitation if breathing or heartbeat stops.
- Get the casualty to hospital as soon as possible (unless the casualty has simply fainted).

Exercise 4.24

Burns and Scalds

Burns are generally caused by dry heat, electricity, friction, or corrosive chemicals. Scalds are caused by moist heat (e.g., boiling water). The pain may be intense, especially with superficial burns. There is usually redness, and blistering occurs later. In addition, there is usually a great deal of shock.

Following are guidelines for treating burns and scalds:

- Immerse the injured area in cold water, or place under slowly running cold water for at least 10 minutes. This decreases the spread of heat and alleviates pain.
- Remove anything that constricts (e.g., rings, clothes, shoes) before the burned area begins to swell.
- Gently remove any clothing that has been soaked in boiling water. Burnt clothing has been sterilised and does not need to be removed.
- Lay the casualty down, and treat for shock.
- Cover the injured part with a clean, dry dressing.
- Give small amounts of cold drinks at frequent intervals if the person is conscious.
- Arrange for immediate removal to hospital for all but the most minor burns.
- Do not apply lotions or ointments.
- Do not prick blisters.
- Do not breathe over, cough over, or touch burned areas.

Bleeding

Major bleeding requires immediate treatment to save the person's life. External bleeding is easy to see, but internal bleeding may only show itself as the signs and symptoms of shock. The aim is to control the bleeding and to keep the wound free of infection. Following are guidelines for treatment:

- Uncover the wound, and check for foreign objects. Do not touch any foreign object that is firmly embedded in a wound. Never pull out an object that has created a puncture wound (e.g., a knife).

- If there are no foreign bodies, apply direct pressure to the wound with the finger and/or hand, preferably over a sterile dressing.

- If the wound is large, squeeze the edges together to try to stop the bleeding.

- Lay the casualty down, and treat for shock.

- If the wound is on a limb and there is no fracture, keep the limb raised.

- Place a sterile, unmedicated dressing over the wound, and secure it firmly with a bandage.

- If the bleeding continues, apply additional dressings on top of the original dressing.

- If direct pressure does not stop the bleeding or if there is an embedded foreign body, use indirect pressure before continuing. To apply indirect pressure, press on the main artery that supplies blood to the limb (e.g., the brachial pressure point on the inside of the upper arm).

- Do not apply indirect pressure for more than 15 minutes at a time, and do not apply a tourniquet.

- Remove the person to hospital for treatment for all but the most minor cuts.

Exercise 4.25

Choking

Clutching the throat is the universal sign for choking. When choking occurs, bend the person forward and give two or three hard slaps between the shoulder blades. Repeat if necessary. If the person is still choking, proceed with the **Heimlich manoeuvre**.

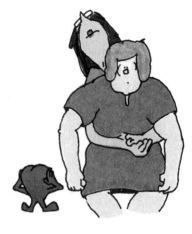

Procedure for a conscious person:

1. Stand behind the person; slide your arms under the choking person's arms and wrap them around the waist.

2. Make a fist, and place it against the person's abdomen—below the rib cage and above the navel, being careful not to touch the sternum (centre breast bone).

3. Using your free hand, apply pressure against your fist with an inward and upward thrust.

4. Give four rapid thrusts, and repeat the procedure if necessary. The abdominal thrusts dislodge the obstruction upward and out from the airway so the person can spit it out.

Procedure for an unconscious person:

When a person loses consciousness from choking, the neck muscles may relax enough that the object no longer completely obstructs the airway. You may be able to remove the obstruction by scooping it out with your fingers.

If the airway is still blocked, follow these steps:

1. Call for emergency help.

2. Place the casualty onto his or her back.

3. Open the airway by tilting the head back and lifting the chin.

4. Check for breathing.

5. If there is no breathing, open the mouth to see if you can scoop the obstruction out with your fingers.

6. If the airway is still blocked, kneel beside or straddle the person at hip level.

7. Place the heel of your hand on the person's abdomen below the rib cage, with your fingers pointing towards the person's chest. Place your free hand over the positioned hand.

8. Position your shoulders over the casualty's abdomen, and thrust your hands inwards and upwards.

9. Give 6 to 10 rapid thrusts.

10. Check to see if the obstruction has been dislodged so that you can remove it from the mouth/throat.

11. Repeat steps 6 to 11, if necessary.

12. After the obstruction has been removed, if the person does not breathe or if the heart has stopped, start cardiopulmonary resuscitation.

Exercise 4.26

Cardiopulmonary Resuscitation

Cardiopulmonary resuscitation (CPR) training teaches valuable life-saving skills. The procedure uses mouth-to-mouth resuscitation and chest compression when the heart and/or the lungs have stopped working. Quick action is critical. CPR must begin as soon as the heart stops in order to prevent brain and internal organ damage.

Only fully trained people should administer CPR. If you have not already attended a course on CPR, you should attend a class as soon as possible.

The following information is NOT a CPR course. It is intended as an overview of the adult basic life-support guidelines for those who have completed CPR training. In this scenario, it will be assumed that you are alone and have found the casualty unresponsive to stimuli.

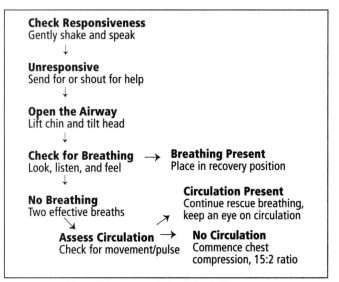

Flow Diagram of Basic Life Support

Following are CPR steps:

1. If possible, leave the victim in the position in which you found him or her. Open the airway by lifting the chin and tilting the head.

2. If this is difficult because of the position, turn the casualty onto the back. If a neck injury is suspected, try to avoid tilting the head.

3. If there is still no response, check for breathing (an occasional gasp should not be interpreted as breathing).

   · **Look** for chest movements.

   · **Listen** by putting your ear near the casualty's nose and mouth.

   · **Feel** for breath on your cheek.

4. Allow up to 10 seconds before deciding the casualty is not breathing. If breathing starts, put the casualty in the recovery position. Send for help if you have not already had the chance to do so, and reassess regularly.

5. If the casualty does not start breathing, if possible send someone for help and start rescue breathing. If you are on your own and cannot send someone for help, follow these guidelines:

   • If the casualty has been subject to trauma or drowning, or is an infant or child, this is usually due to primary respiratory arrest. In this case, give rescue breaths for about one minute (approximately 10 breaths) before reassessment; and, if the person starts breathing, go for help.

   • If the casualty does not fall into the above category, the cause of collapse is much more likely to be cardiac in origin, and defibrillation is the key to survival. Therefore, leave the casualty as soon as you have established that he or she is not breathing (rather than give rescue breaths) in order to get help. The casualty needs advanced life support.

6. Use precautions to prevent infection, if possible. (Remember, you are potentially at risk from *all* people.)

7. Tilt the head back by lifting the neck. Inspect the mouth for any obvious obstruction. Leave well-fitting dentures in place.

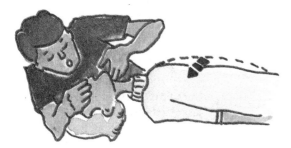

8. Pinch the nose closed to prevent air from escaping from the nostrils, and cover the casualty's mouth completely with your mouth.

9. Blow into the person's mouth until you see the chest rise and fall. A breath volume of 400-500 cc is sufficient to provide adequate ventilation. Take about 1 1/2-2 seconds to breathe air into the casualty, resulting in an inflation/exhalation cycle of about 3-4 seconds.

10. After you have delivered two effective breaths of rescue breathing, assess the casualty for signs of circulation. Take no longer than 10 seconds to do this.

11. Look for movement such as swallowing or breathing.

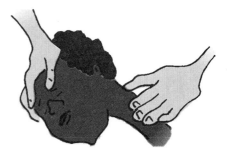

12. Check the carotid pulse at the side of the neck. If the pulse is present, continue rescue breathing if necessary. Re-check for signs of circulation every minute, taking no longer than 10 seconds each time. If the casualty starts to breathe, but remains unconscious, put the person into the recovery position.

13. If there is no pulse, or if you are not sure, commence chest compressions—about 100 per minute.

   • Ensure that the casualty is lying on a firm surface.

   • Locate the lower end of the sternum, and place the heel of the hand over the end portion of the casualty's sternum.

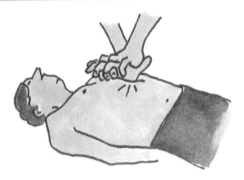

- Then place the heel of your other hand over the top of the first hand to increase leverage.

- Use the heels of your hands to compress the chest.

14. Combine chest compression with rescue breathing at a rate of 15:2 if you are alone (or 5:1 if there are two of you). Only check the pulse again if the casualty takes a spontaneous breath. Take no longer than 10 seconds to do this.

15. Continue resuscitation until the casualty shows signs of life or until qualified help arrives.

Exercise 4.27

Diabetes Mellitus

Diabetes mellitus is a medical condition where a person cannot produce enough insulin. Insulin is the hormone produced by the pancreas to help the body break down and convert sugars and starches into energy. Two complications of diabetes which require prompt attention are hyperglycaemia and hypoglycaemia.

Hyperglycaemia (diabetic coma) is the result of too little insulin or too much sugar. It occurs when blood sugar levels are high and there is an acidosis due to ketones being present in the blood. Although the onset of this condition is gradual, it is life-threatening and requires immediate medical care.

Early signs of hyperglycaemia:

- thirst
- abdominal pain
- nausea
- drowsiness
- increased urination

Later signs of hyperglycaemia:

- heavy breathing
- breath smells of pear drops
- dry skin
- flushed face
- loss of consciousness

Stay with the person to offer reassurance until the ambulance arrives to take him or her to hospital for treatment. At hospital, insulin is given to reduce the blood sugar, and sodium bicarbonate solution (an alkali) is given to counteract the acidosis and dehydration.

Hypoglycaemia (insulin shock) is the result of too much insulin or too little sugar. The onset of this condition is very quick as the lowered blood sugar affects the functioning of the brain.

Signs of hypoglycaemia:

- lethargy, weakness, dizziness
- hunger
- unconsciousness
- confusion or bad temperedness
- sweating

Treatment includes giving glucose orally, as quickly as possible, before the person loses consciousness. In severe cases where the person loses consciousness, glucose is injected intravenously (into a vein) by a doctor. Stay with the person and offer reassurance until he or she recovers. This should happen very quickly after the glucose has been administered. Report hypoglycaemic attacks to the person-in-charge, and accurately record details of the attack (date, time, symptoms, speed of recovery, etc.).

If you are unsure whether a person who has diabetes mellitus is having a hypoglycaemic or hyperglycaemic attack, give the person glucose. If it is hypoglycaemia, recovery will happen very quickly. If it is hyperglycaemia, no harm will be done because it is the acidosis in hyperglycaemia that causes the major problems, not the raised blood sugar.

Exercise 4.28 🖊

Seizures

A seizure (fit) occurs when normal brain cell activity is interrupted by abnormal discharges of electricity within the brain. Seizures can happen to anyone. They are often caused by the following:

- tumours
- stroke
- chemical imbalance
- head injury
- infection and fever

Sometimes no cause can be found. When a person has seizures, even when they occur only occasionally, the person is said to have epilepsy.

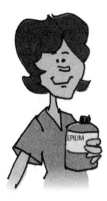

The main treatment for epilepsy is medication (e.g., Epilim). Medication strengthens a person's resistance to seizures. It is important that people who suffer from epilepsy take their medication regularly, as prescribed. Medication completely controls epilepsy for some people; for others, seizures are kept to a minimum.

Generalised absence (petit mal) seizures are characterised by the person looking blank and staring. There may be slight blinking or twitching. This type of seizure lasts for only a few seconds. Afterwards the person continues as normal, as if nothing has happened, unaware of the seizure.

Complex partial (psychomotor) seizures may start with an "aura" or warning (e.g., seeing flashing lights or having a horrible taste in the mouth). The person appears confused or distracted and may repeat a series of movements (e.g., plucking at clothes).

Generalised tonic-clonic (grand mal) seizures tend to have a common sequence of events. However, not all tonic-clonic seizures will exactly follow the sequence. This type of seizure can last for several minutes. It tends to be noisy and is very frightening for onlookers. There may be an aura followed by staring, followed by a stiffening of the body, which usually results in the person falling to the ground. The person may cry out. There may be a blue colour around the mouth and extremities. Eventually the person commences convulsions (jerking movements). As these fade away, breathing restarts and normal colour returns. There is often foaming at the mouth, and this can be blood-flecked. Occasionally, there is incontinence. The person may appear to sleep for a short while before regaining consciousness.

Exercise 4.29 🖊

Status epilepticus occurs when a person has repeated tonic-clonic seizures without recovering consciousness. This is a medical emergency. The person may die without prompt medical attention.

Do whatever is necessary to protect the person from injury during a seizure. Do not try to restrain the person. Never pry the mouth open, and do not insert anything into the mouth.

To care for tonic-clonic seizures, do whatever is necessary to protect the person from injury. Try to support the person if he or she falls to the floor (be careful not to injure your back). If the person has not fallen to the floor, lay the person down. Move furniture and equipment out of the way to prevent injury during the convulsion stage of the seizure. Do not leave the person alone during the seizure.

If the person is in bed and there are side rails, pad the rails with blankets or soft foam. Take care to protect the person's head from injury during a seizure. If possible, turn the head to one side to prevent choking.

If the seizure occurs in a care facility, if appropriate, help the person to bed, report all seizures to the person-in-charge, and chart the seizure, recording all relevant details (e.g., date, time, description of the seizure, length of recovery).

After a tonic-clonic seizure, be aware that the person will not remember the seizure. Provide reassurance, and help the person to his or her feet. Observe closely in case the person is confused or has another seizure.

Electrocution

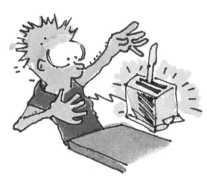

Electrical injuries can kill or cause a wide range of injuries, including severe burns and heart stoppage. Most electrical accidents involve household appliances, and lighting circuits can have the same effect. The extent of injuries usually depends on the strength of the electrical current, how long the victim was exposed, and amount of insulation (e.g., whether the victim was wearing rubber-soled shoes or standing on a dry surface).

Never approach the victim of an electrical accident until you are sure it is safe. If the casualty is still in contact with the source of electricity, cut off the power supply before you touch the person by turning off the switch or unplugging the appliance.

If you cannot turn off the electricity supply because there are high voltage power lines, do not approach. You can receive a fatal shock up to 20 yards away. If it is household equipment that you cannot turn off and the casualty is still holding the source of electricity, stand on a rubber mat or dry newspaper, and lever the person's hand away using a wooden broom handle.

Once the casualty is safely removed from the electrical source, you can apply first aid. Smother any flames with a blanket or towel. If the casualty has been thrown to the ground by the electrical shock, check for breathing and pulse. Start CPR, if necessary. Then check that there are no fractures, and treat any burns. Electrical burns may be much deeper than their size suggests. Provide reassurance and help as needed.

Exercise 4.30

Chest Pains

Chest pains can occur for a number of reasons. The most common cause of chest pain is angina. Angina is a severe, but temporary, attack of chest pain which is often induced by exercise. A person with chest pains will have a good idea whether the pain is angina or not.

If it is angina, sit or lay the person down and help the person take a heart tablet (that angina sufferers usually have with them). The tablet is usually placed under the tongue and allowed to dissolve. Once the person is at rest, the angina attack should soon disappear.

Chest pain could signal a heart attack. A heart attack is a potentially fatal reduction in blood supply to the heart. Signs include severe shock, severe and constricting chest pain, sometimes radiating down the arm and neck (usually the left side). There may be shortness of breath, weak and irregular pulse, and unconsciousness.

First aid for a heart attack:

- Provide reassurance.

- Put the casualty into the most comfortable position. This is usually sitting up (the best position to help breathing).

- Get medical attention as quickly as possible as the casualty needs urgent treatment.

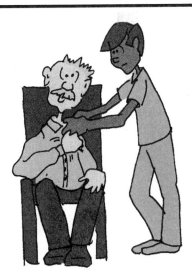

- Loosen tight clothing at the neck, chest, and waist, and encourage deep breathing.

- If the casualty becomes unconscious, check the pulse and respirations. Commence CPR if there is no pulse or respiration.

Exercise 4.31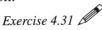

Fractures

A fracture is a cracked or broken bone. There are two main causes of fracture—direct force (e.g., from a kick to the shin), and indirect force (e.g., falling on an outstretched hand and fracturing the collar bone). The casualty may have heard the bone break. Crepitus (i.e., the sound of two broken ends of bone grating together) can sometimes be heard . The casualty will probably not be able to use the affected part of the body, or it will be very painful to do so. The area of skin over the fracture will usually be swollen and bruised. The body part may be in an unnatural position or look different than the same body part on the other side of the body.

- **Simple fractures:** The skin is unbroken, but there may be heavy bruising.

- **Complicated fractures:** There is damage to surrounding tissues (e.g., when a fractured pelvis punctures the bladder).

- **Compound fractures:** The bone protrudes through the skin, or the skin is lacerated above the fracture leaving an opening for micro-organisms to enter.

- **Greenstick fractures:** The bone is bent and may half break. These fractures occur in children.

Treat all bone injuries as fractures until diagnosis proves otherwise. Move the casualty as little as possible. Make the person as comfortable as possible, handling with great care so that you do not increase injury, pain, and shock.

Gently remove clothing from any open wound over the break, and cover with a clean dressing. If a bone protrudes, pack around it so that the bandage used to hold the dressing does not press directly onto the bone.

Immobilise the fracture if possible. There are many different ways of immobilising the different fractures. For example, put a broken arm in a sling or immobilise a broken leg by using the other leg as a splint. Remember to pad between bony prominences. Treat for shock, provide reassurance, and get the casualty to hospital as quickly as possible. Do not give the person anything to eat or drink.

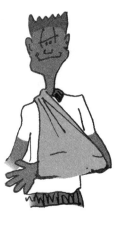

Exercise 4.32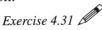

Poisoning

Poison is a substance which, if taken into the body in sufficient quantity, can cause temporary or permanent damage. Poisons tend to be swallowed, inhaled, absorbed through the skin, or injected. Poisoning is often accidental (e.g., a child who drinks bleach), but it can also be deliberate (e.g., a person who is trying to commit suicide).

The signs and symptoms of poisoning vary greatly, depending on the poison, the method of entry, and the amount taken. Once in the body, the poison finds its way into the bloodstream where it is swiftly taken to all parts of the body.

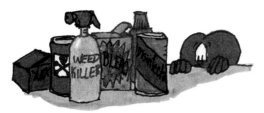

A conscious casualty or onlooker may tell you that poisoning has occurred. When the casualty is unconscious, other features (such as a fume-filled room or empty tablet bottles) may tell you what you need to know.

If the casualty is conscious, ensure an open airway and monitor breathing and circulation. If the casualty is unconscious, place in the recovery position.

To prevent further injury from poisons, follow these guidelines:

- **Swallowed poisons**: Do not attempt to induce vomiting as this may harm the casualty further. If the casualty's lips are burned by corrosive substances, give frequent sips of cold water or milk.
- **Inhaled poisons**: Remove the casualty from danger into the fresh air. At work, do not enter gas-filled rooms unless you are authorised and properly equipped to do so.

- **Absorbed poisons**: Flush away any residual chemicals on the skin, making sure that you do not get any on your skin.
- Where appropriate, try to identify the poison.
- Obtain appropriate medical attention.

Exercise 4.33 ✎

Summary

The people in your care depend on you for their health, safety, and security. Your responsibilities include monitoring and maintaining each client's safety and security in the care environment. Vital skills for care support workers include preventing accidents, minimising risks, and handling emergencies.

Two important principles for maintaining your own health and safety (as well as the clients') are manual handling and infection control. Always follow safe manual handling procedures, and use the available manual handling equipment. Ensure that you understand and adhere to the principles of infection control, especially the Universal Precautions.

Check Your Knowledge and Understanding

1. Jimmy, a resident on your day care unit, appears to be missing. He has wandered off the unit before and has put himself in danger. What should you do?

   a) Immediately implement the missing person procedure.

   b) Give him another hour to see if he wanders back to the unit on his own.

   c) Search the building thoroughly, and then search the grounds and local areas.

   d) Contact the police.

2. You smell burning at work one day, although you cannot see a fire or any smoke. What would you do?

   a) Ignore the smell of burning as it may be coming from outside the building.

   b) Carry out a more thorough search for the source of the smell.

   c) Immediately raise the alarm and evacuate the building.

   d) Walk around the building to check that the fire extinguishers are all in working order.

3. You need to move a partially mobile person up in bed. Another carer who is a new member of staff comes to help you and states that she has not yet done the manual handling course, but she is willing to try a "drag lift." What would you do?

   a) Go ahead and use the drag lift because there is nobody else available to help you at the moment.

   b) Fetch a handling sling and show the new carer how to move the client up the bed.

   c) Lift the person up in bed by yourself.

   d) Gently explain that someone who has not yet completed the manual handling course should not be involved in the lifting and moving of clients. Then wait until somebody else is available to help you.

4. An intravenous drug user, who is known to be HIV positive, is attending your day centre. Several of your colleagues claim that they are scared of catching AIDS. What would you do?

   a) Say, "I can understand your fears, but there is nothing you can do to stop this person attending the day centre."

   b) Suggest that your colleagues book in for an AIDS workshop.

   c) Advise them to see the day centre manager to express their fears and pick up copies of the AIDS leaflets.

   d) Tell them to stop being silly as they cannot catch AIDS from this person unless they have intimate sexual contact.

5. Someone comes to you who has just sustained a nasty burn to his hand from touching the steam iron. What would you do?

   a) Immediately apply a clean, dry dressing to prevent infection, after removing the person's rings in case the fingers blister.

b) Immediately apply some antiseptic cream after removing the rings, but before applying the dressing.

c) Immediately put the person's hand under a slow-running tap, and gently slip the rings off the person's fingers.

d) Prick the blisters as they start to form, and then apply a clean, dry dressing.

6. A diabetic client, who is suffering from an ear infection, claims to be feeling unwell. He appears to be a bit confused and is sweating. What would you do?

a) Quickly put a couple of glucose sweets into the person's mouth.

b) Call for the doctor.

c) Ask him to go to bed, and offer him an aspirin, saying you will check up on him later to see if he is any better.

d) Advise the client to give himself more insulin.

Module 5

Providing Physical Comfort and Enabling Movement

Maximise physical comfort and enable others to move safely.

Objectives:

- Describe the different types of pain and how pain should be assessed.
- Outline a range of treatments for acute and chronic pain.
- Ensure that a client can achieve rest.
- Describe how to manage insomnia.
- Outline how the dangers to client and carer can be minimised during manual handling.
- Demonstrate a range of techniques that are used for the manual handling of clients.
- Demonstrate the correct usage of a variety of manual handling aids.
- Describe the problems caused by immobility.
- Demonstrate how to undertake passive and active exercises with clients.
- Outline how mobility aids can be maintained and safely used by clients.
- Explain how pressure sores can be prevented.
- Demonstrate the correct use of pressure-relieving equipment.

Module 5 Introduction

Module 5 relates to three units of the level 2 NVQ/SVQ Award in Care:

Unit Z19: **Enable clients to achieve physical comfort** is an option group B unit. It consists of two elements of competence:

- Z19.1 Assist in minimising client pain and discomfort.

- Z19.2 Assist in providing conditions to meet clients' need for rest.

Unit Z7: **Contribute to the movement and handling of clients to maximise their physical comfort** is an option group B unit. It consists of three elements of competence:

- Z7.1 Prepare clients and environments for moving and handling.

- Z7.2 Assist clients to move from one position to another.

- Z7.3 Assist clients to prevent and minimise the adverse effects of pressure.

Unit Z6: **Enable clients to maintain and improve their mobility through exercise and the use of mobility appliances** is an option group B unit. It consists of two elements of competence:

- Z6.1 Enable clients to exercise.

- Z6.2 Assist clients to use mobility appliances.

Part 1: Enabling Others to Achieve Physical Comfort (Z19)

Promote well-being by enabling others to rest and be pain-free.

When an individual is suffering from pain in the short or long term, life can be rather unpleasant. Your goal must be to minimise, or get rid of, the client's pain.

There are many definitions of pain. One example is "a complex phenomenon which consists of an unpleasant sensory and emotional experience associated with actual or potential tissue damage."

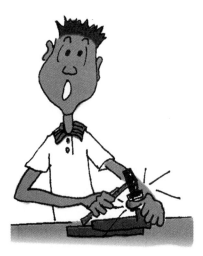

Another definition describes pain as "what the client says it is in terms of where it is, what type it is, and how much it hurts." This is a useful definition because there is only one person who can have a clear idea of the nature of the pain that is being felt—the client.

Superficial pain usually involves the skin or mucous membranes of the body. There are many pain receptors in these areas of the body which can be activated by a range of stimuli—mechanical, electrical, chemical, or thermal. The pain is described as bright, pricking, burning, and is usually localised.

Deep pain originates from somewhere within the body, but may not be so localised as superficial pain. Deep pain usually has an aching quality.

Referred pain is pain that is felt at a site other than that where the nerve receptors have been stimulated (e.g., the pain of a heart attack may result in referred pain in the left shoulder and arm).

Acute pain has a sudden onset and a foreseeable end. It is accompanied by a stress or anxiety reaction in the client caused by the release of adrenaline into the body. This results in dilation of the pupils and an increased pulse and respiration rate. Acute pain is regularly seen in casualty departments and surgical wards.

Chronic pain is an ongoing, long-term (usually more than six months) problem that needs to be managed. It tends to affect the lifestyles of sufferers. Chronic pain is often accompanied by sleep disturbances, loss of appetite and sex drive, constipation, a preoccupation with the illness and the pain, changes in personality, and an inability to work.

Exercise 5.1 ✎

An individual's safety is severely compromised if he or she cannot feel pain. Acute pain has a protective role, warning an individual of actual or potential tissue damage and stimulating movement away from the source of harm. The benefits of chronic pain are less easy to determine, but may relate to forcing an individual to rest a damaged part of the body until it has time to recover.

The gate control theory of pain attempts to explain the variations in the perception of pain felt by different individuals who have been subject to the same pain stimulus. In its simplest form, the theory proposes that there is a "gate" in the spinal cord through which nerve impulses have to travel so that they can be interpreted by the brain. When the gate is open, the pain impulses can pass through easily, and when the gate is closed, none can pass through.

It is thought that the amount of opening of the gate is influenced by the strength of the pain signal and a number of psychological factors. This theory is useful because it emphasises the fact that the level of pain perceived by a client is not just dependent on the strength of the pain signal received from the affected part of the body.

The gate control theory can be highlighted by the following example. Members of the armed forces may not report pain because they are highly relieved to be away from the field of battle and to be alive. However, a civilian casualty of a car accident with the same injuries may report feeling a lot of pain, especially if the accident was someone else's fault and the person is feeling resentful about being hurt.

Therefore, there is no predictable relationship between pain and injury. Each person's pain experience is modified by a number of factors which include pain tolerance, personality, mood, level of perceived stress, life experiences, culture, etc.

Exercise 5.2 ✎

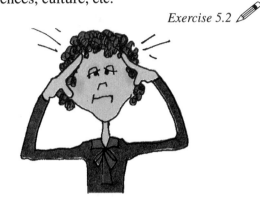

Some care workers think that they know best in terms of the client's pain—the type of pain and how intense it is. This is because they may feel uneasy about believing the client's statement of feeling pain. Since the care worker has no objective evidence about the type and level of pain perceived by the client, he or she should rely solely on information about the pain provided by the client. This may occasionally mean that you provide pain relief for a malingerer, which is better than not providing pain relief for a client who really needs it.

Usually, the clients who are more emotional will feel the most pain. Sometimes clients can adapt to pain so that it is very difficult for a care worker to notice if the client is suffering. An example here is where a client commences knitting or watching television as a distraction. Because the client is occupied, he or she does not appear to be in pain. However, you simply cannot assume that the pain is not there just because the client is not showing any obvious symptoms.

A further problem is where a client is afraid or embarrassed to report that he or she is in pain. In addition, special care has to be taken for those clients who physically cannot express the amount of pain they have because of communication difficulties, mental health problems, etc.

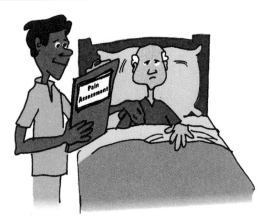

Pain Assessment

Because pain is a subjective experience for the client, it is the responsibility of the care support worker and other members of the care team to recognise that a client is suffering from pain and to report these facts to an appropriate authority for further action. Remember that pain is assessed *with* the client, not *on* the client.

The signs and symptoms that may indicate that a client is suffering from pain include the following:

- The client says he or she is in pain.

- The client has an elevated blood pressure, pulse rate, and respiration rate.

- The client is perspiring more than usual.

- The client is writhing about, or there is increased restlessness.

- Because pain is fatiguing, the client may simply be quieter than usual and is lying still because he or she is too tired to do otherwise.

- The client exhibits other associated symptoms (e.g., vomiting, mobility difficulties).

Exercise 5.3 ✎

Each individual client who is suffering from pain should have the pain assessed. This can vary from asking the client (e.g., "Do you have any pain at the moment, Mr. Smith?") to the use of a pain assess-

ment chart which allows a more accurate assessment of the client's pain.

If no pain assessment forms are available, you can construct your own. Make up a simple body chart by drawing the outline of the front and back views of the human body. The client can then mark the site of pain with a pen or pencil. The level of pain can be identified by asking the client to place a cross on a scale of 1 to 10.

0 ———————————————————— 10

No pain   The worst pain I can possibly imagine

Ask the client about the quality or type of pain (e.g., stabbing, burning, aching) and the pattern of pain (e.g., continuous, comes and goes, slowly increasing).

There are no set rules for how often a client's pain should be assessed. The assessment should be often enough to monitor the effectiveness of pain therapies that are being used and to ensure that the client's pain is controlled (e.g., every two hours for a client who has returned to a hospital ward after having an operation, three times a day for a client who is suffering from arthritis).

Exercise 5.4 ✎

Pain Therapies

Everyone experiences pain or discomfort at times. You should aim to prevent or reduce pain and discomfort as much as possible. No client should be allowed to suffer any longer than necessary. Individual beliefs and cultural background often affect the way a person prefers to handle pain or discomfort.

There are a number of different treatments or therapies that can be used to manage a client's pain. The acceptability of these different pain therapies to the client will depend on the client's culture and background. In most circumstances, it is appropriate to manage a client's pain by using a combination of at least two of the following approaches—physical, pharmacological, and psychological. Following are examples of pain treatments.

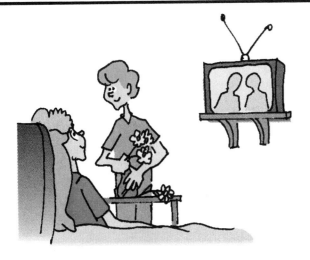

Distraction is a non-invasive pain therapy. It occurs when the client is encouraged to focus attention on events other than the pain. Sometimes this can occur naturally (e.g., when the client is reading or watching the television). Alternatively, the care worker can plan a number of distractions with the client. Distraction can increase a client's tolerance to pain, and sometimes it decreases the intensity of the pain as the pain ceases to be the client's focus of attention. Distraction is often used for interim pain relief until another form of analgesia takes effect.

Exercise 5.5 🖉

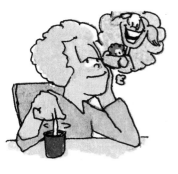

Imagery is a type of distraction that focuses on personal thoughts. When the client is using imagery, he or she is concentrating very hard on thoughts rather than on the pain. Imagery usually involves the use of progressive relaxation techniques followed by the imagining of idyllic scenes (e.g., thinking of the "good old days").

Relaxation techniques are another type of non-invasive pain therapy. They are used to produce freedom from mental and physical anxiety and stress. There are several techniques available (e.g., meditation, yoga, mild to moderate exercise, progressive relaxation exercises, massage, hypnosis). They all require the client's participation. As with distraction and imagery, they can be taught to the client for use on him/herself.

Exercise 5.6 🖉

Transcutaneous electric nerve stimulation (TENS) is used for the relief of both acute and chronic pain. The system basically consists of a battery-powered electronic pulse generator which is connected to four wires (electrodes) that are attached to the skin in an area served by the same nerves as the source of pain. The stimulation of the electric current is felt by the client as a tingling or buzzing sensation. This can be adjusted by increasing or decreasing the electric current until the client achieves pain relief. TENS works by bombarding the pain nerve pathways with non-painful stimuli at the same level in the spinal cord that it is receiving pain impulses from the painful part of the body.

Acupuncture is a treatment where fine needles are pushed into the skin at various points in the body called meridians in order to achieve specific physical effects. The place where the needles are inserted may be close to the point of pain or quite far away. The needles can be rotated or stimulated by electricity to increase their effect. A similar effect can be achieved by the use of massage on pressure points, referred to as *acupressure*.

Analgesics are a common method of pain relief. They are usually given in the form of a tablet, injection, or suppository. They vary in terms of site of action, side effects, toxicity, and adverse effects (e.g., allergic reactions). Although doctors usually prescribe them, it is important that other care workers take responsibility for their administration and the monitoring of their effectiveness. The need for analgesia must be reported immediately so that medication can be given to the client.

There are two main types of analgesics. *Narcotic* analgesics (e.g., morphine and pethidine) are usually very potent. They act directly on the central nervous system of the body, and they are usually the only effective analgesic for severe pain.

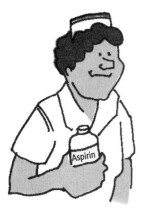

Non-narcotic analgesics (e.g., aspirin, paracetamol, and ibuprofen) are less potent than narcotic drugs. They usually act on the nerves at the site of the problem and are effective for mild to moderate pain. The care support worker is often the person that a client will turn to for pain relief. Make sure that, in your organisation, you know who is allowed, and who is not allowed, to be involved in the administration of medications.

Exercise 5.7 🖋

Clients who are suffering from pain or discomfort sometimes encounter a number of problems within care environments. Pain can be suffered unnecessarily by clients when there is a delay in providing pain relief (e.g., due to a shortage of qualified care staff, when care staff only provide analgesia during drug rounds).

In a small number of care environments, care workers can act as judge and jury by deciding if the pain is reasonable, timely, and expected in terms of the client's condition and, therefore, worthy of receiving pain relief. Or, care staff may only provide pain relief in return for good client behaviour.

Even when pain relief has been prescribed and is available, the client may not be aware that analgesia is available unless this has been carefully explained. The client may not want to trouble the care workers if they appear busy or uncaring. If a client's pain is not monitored on an ongoing basis, the care staff may not be aware of the client's pain.

Clients who are receiving analgesic drugs may develop a *psychological dependence* on the drug. That is, the clients feel the need to continue taking the drugs, whether or not the drugs are needed.

Sometimes clients develop a *physical dependence* with addictive drugs. Withdrawal of the drugs can make them feel very ill. Also a drug tolerance may develop, and increasing amounts of drugs will be needed to achieve the same clinical effects.

Problems of communication between different care professionals can result in disagreement on the best way to manage the pain. The client may be given conflicting information/advice about the problem.

Ongoing pain may result in a client becoming overly anxious and depressed. This may make it even more difficult for the client to get on with his or her life.

Exercise 5.8 🖋

Pain Management

Ensure that you are clear about your expected role in relation to the minimising of clients' pain and discomfort. Find out from the clients how they would normally manage pain. You can then involve the clients in planning ways to manage their problems, and their views can be utilised in agreeing their plans of care.

The provisions that have been made for the management of each client's pain should be carefully and clearly explained to the client. If nothing else, this makes it clear that the care staff are interested in each client as a person and in each client's 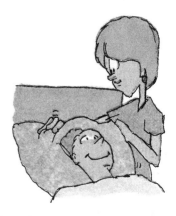 well-being. This knowledge alone can reduce anxiety and the subsequent levels of pain that are perceived by the client.

Provide clients with all necessary information about the plan of pain management in a manner and at a level and pace that is appropriate for them. If a client uses homeopathic or homely remedies for the management of pain, these should be continued unless they are likely to adversely affect the treatment that has been prescribed, or they are unacceptable to the care environment (e.g., illegal drugs, large quantities of alcohol).

Encourage the client to express feelings of pain by reporting discomfort to one of the care staff. If monitoring pain or discomfort is part of the plan of care, maintain accurate records of levels of pain, treatments, and response to treatments.

The emphasis should be on *pain control*, rather than pain relief. That is, the client should be free from the peaks of pain that occur as the effects of a pain relief treatment wear off. Ensure that the client is comfortable in terms of warmth, position, appropriate lighting and ventilation, and ensure that the client is moved with care. Pain is fatiguing, which in itself can increase a client's perception of pain and lead to delays in recovery and rehabilitation. Therefore, it is important to ensure that the client receives prompt pain relief and gets adequate rest.

Offer support to anyone who is disturbed or upset by the client's pain or discomfort. Seek advice from an appropriate person if you have any problems in managing a client's pain or discomfort.

Exercise 5.9

Rest

People have different requirements for sleep and rest, which are dependent on age, level of activity, cultural norms, etc. Some people appear to be always "on the go," keeping themselves busy throughout the day, and requiring no more than four or five hours sleep at night. At the other end of the scale are those who require regular rest periods throughout the day which can include a siesta and at least 10 hours of sleep each night. Most people fall between the two extremes.

It is important that clients meet their personal needs for rest. There are a number of illnesses where an increased amount of rest and sleep is essential for the healing process. When an individual does not get enough rest, health problems are likely to develop. The discomfort caused by an illness may prevent the client from achieving adequate rest and sleep. The individual's ability to rest and sleep can be affected by a number of different factors (e.g., physical pain, psychological stress, and environmental noise). Report any areas of concern to the person-in-charge.

Exercise 5.10

Provide conditions that are suitable for rest. Use appropriate, relaxed behaviour, movements, and tone of voice to encourage rest and relaxation. Talk to the client and/or the family to find out the client's normal pattern of resting throughout the day. Do not try and guess the client's rest requirements, and do not dictate when the client is expected to rest.

The provisions that are generally made for clients to rest within a care environment should be carefully explained to clients in a manner and at a pace and level that they can understand. This can form the basis for negotiating times for rest within the client's plan of care.

Observe the client for signs of tiredness (e.g., droopy eyelids, limp body posture) so that you can mention to the client that he or she appears tired, and then suggest a period of rest. Encourage the client to tell you when he or she needs to rest.

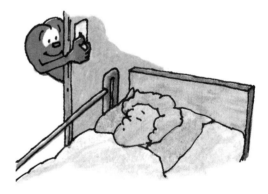

Adjust light, noise, heat, and ventilation as much as possible to meet the client's requirements, without upsetting any other clients who are in the same environment. You cannot please everybody, and an element of compromise may be necessary. It may be necessary to remove the client to an environment where he or she can rest in peace and quiet.

Assist the client into a comfortable position, consistent with the plan of care. If the client's condition requires sitting or lying in an unfamiliar position, you may have to try different positions until the most comfortable one is found.

Enable the client to undertake any usual pre-rest routines or activities (e.g., read a book, do some knitting, have a cup of tea, undertake yoga or relaxation exercises). Ensure that the activity does not adversely affect the treatment that has been prescribed or is unacceptable to the care environment (e.g., illegal drugs, large quantities of alcohol).

If the client requires any care (e.g., using the toilet, treatments, or medications), either provide the care before the client rests, or arrange for the care after the client has rested. If possible, ensure that the client is not unnecessarily disturbed whilst resting by other clients, friends or relatives, or by care workers (e.g., providing unwanted cups of tea). If necessary, provide appropriate reminders to others to keep noise and disturbance to a minimum.

If monitoring the client's rest is part of the plan of care, maintain accurate, legible, and complete records. Seek advice if you are having difficulties in promoting rest for an individual client or group of clients.

Exercise 5.11 🖉

Insomnia

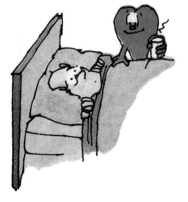

Insomnia is a disorder of initiating and maintaining sleep. Sleep is an important process to remedy the "wear and tear" of the waking hours. Before there is any attempt made at treating insomnia, a thorough assessment of the causes is essential. Following are some factors that can affect an individual's ability to sleep:

- Illness, coughing, or pain
- Hunger or thirst
- Worrying or thinking
- The sleep environment (e.g., comfort of the bed or positioning, level of temperature or lighting, amount of noise)
- Stimulation (e.g., caffeine)
- The need to use the toilet
- Level of tiredness
- Interrupted pre-sleep routine

Exercise 5.12 🖉

Guidelines for managing insomnia are very similar to those used for promoting rest, but they should focus on the causes of the insomnia. A client's normal sleeping pattern needs to be considered (e.g., a night shift worker may find it very difficult to settle into a pattern of regular nighttime sleeping).

A pre-sleep routine within the plan of care can be especially important for tackling insomnia. If a client uses homeopathic or homely remedies as part of the routine, these should be continued unless they are likely to adversely affect the treatment that has been prescribed or they are unacceptable to the care environment (e.g., illegal drugs, large quantities of alcohol).

Drinking caffeinated coffee and tea, especially in the evening, should be avoided. Caffeine is a stimulant and may keep the client awake. Too many fluids in the couple of hours prior to going to sleep may cause nocturia (the need to urinate during the night).

A new bed or freshly laundered bed clothes or pillows may promote sleep. Unless absolutely necessary, discourage naps during the day so that the client is sufficiently tired to go to sleep at night. Bear in mind that disturbing a client during the night (e.g., for pressure area care, treatment) can significantly reduce the total amount of sleep that a client achieves each night.

For some clients, perfect quiet and darkness are required for sleep. Unfortunately, this is not achievable in some care areas (e.g., an acute care hospital ward, when other clients are not quiet during the night). The best that can be achieved is to reduce the light and noise to a minimum (e.g., turning the lights down, whispering instead of talking, wearing soft heeled shoes, making sure that the wheels of trolleys do not squeak). As a last resort, a doctor may prescribe medication to help relaxation or induce sleep.

Take care when monitoring and recording a client's sleep patterns. It is not uncommon for the care report to say that a client has slept all night whilst the patient reports "hardly sleeping a wink" because of discomfort or pain. Ensure that your reports are accurate, legible, and complete. If you have any concerns in relation to the sleep patterns of clients or in relation to the appropriateness of the environment for sleep, report your concerns to the person-in-charge.

Exercise 5.13

Part 2: Enabling Others to Move (Z7.1/2)

Safely undertake manual handling tasks.

Manual handling procedures involve both hazards and risks. A hazard can be defined as something which may cause harm. Risk is an expression of the probability of the harm or injury occurring. Hazards and risks are present for both care workers and clients involved in manual handling.

The stresses exerted on the spine during manual handling tasks are mainly the result of the techniques used. The Manual Handling Operations Regulations provide clear guidelines on moving and lifting practice and a framework for risk assessment. You must use only those manual handling techniques and equipment that are sanctioned by your employing organisation.

Exercise 5.14

Information concerning the lifting and moving of clients, and its relationship to personal health and safety, can be found in Module 4, Part 2.

Refer to the table on the right when deciding on whether a lift is safe. The weight capacities are only for lifting in the ideal position, with the load being held close to the lower body of the care worker(s).

Lifting Capacities			
	1 Carer	2 Carers	3 Carers
Men	25 kg (3 st 13 lb)	33.3 kg (5 st 13 lb)	37.5 kg (5 st 12 lb)
Women	16.6 kg (2 st 8 lb)	22.2 kg (3 st 7 lb)	25 kg (3 st 13 lb)

Exercise 5.15

The emphasis is on avoiding manual lifting whenever possible. In the ideal situation, when clients require assistance with mobility, hoists, sliding aids, and handling slings should be made available. An employer who does not make available this kind of equipment and associated training is in conflict with the law, as are the care workers who choose to ignore the equipment. The systems of safe practice for manual handling are implemented locally for everybody's safety and protection.

You are required to adapt the task to suit the environment, the available manual handling aids, and the skills and physical abilities of the individuals undertaking it. The expectation is that all manual handling tasks must be assessed in advance every time the task has to be carried out.

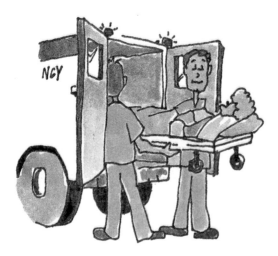

It is essential for you to recognise when a manual handling task is beyond your capabilities. Then you need to be assertive enough to refuse to undertake the task until additional equipment and/or assistance is available. Report the situation to an appropriate member of the care team. Help may be available from a number of sources (e.g., the ambulance service in the community).

Take action to remove or reduce the risk of injury to all participants. The actions and support provided should be consistent with the plan of care and the outcomes of the initial assessment. Where possible, involve the client in the decision making on the level of support that is needed for the move.

Many clients are able to assist the care workers who are moving them. They should be encouraged to do so, as long as it is in ways that are appropriate to their capabilities and health status.

Exercise 5.16

Manual Handling Guidelines

The manual handling task that needs to be achieved should be clearly defined. If necessary, the task should be divided into sub-tasks that can be assessed separately (e.g., from lying on the bed to being sat at the edge of the bed to transfer to a chair). A flowchart, providing guidance on the moving and handling of clients, can be seen on the right.

Exercise 5.17

Does the client need to be moved?	No →	Do not proceed.
↓ Yes		
Is there a care plan for moving this client?	Yes →	Follow the care plan.
↓ No		
Can the client safely move him/herself?	Yes →	Encourage the client to move self.
↓ No		
Can the client help with the move?	Yes →	Allow the client to help as much as possible.
↓ No		
Have you assessed the risks?	No →	Assess the risk before you move the client.
↓ Yes		
Would a lifting aid help?	No →	Is there a technique that you can safely use?
↓ Yes		
Are appropriate lifting aids available?	No →	Do not proceed. Seek advice.
↓ Yes		
Do you know how to use the lifting aids?	No →	Do not proceed. Seek advice.

Is there a technique that you can safely use? No → Seek advice.

Yes → Are there enough trained people available for the move?

Yes ↙

Yes ↘ Implement the move. ←

Flowchart for the Manual Handling of Clients

Check the client's care plan, and assess the needs of the client and any limitations imposed by the care environment or available resources. Use the flow diagram above, and inform all care staff involved in the task. If you are unsure about how to undertake the manual handling task or if you are not sure whether the proposed move or transfer is safe, report your concerns to the person-in-charge. If available, contact your organisation's manual handling coordinator for advice.

With the client's permission, prepare the care area by moving all unnecessary furniture and equipment out of the way. Inform the client what you are about to do, even when the client is unconscious. Your aims are to move the client in ways which minimise pain, discomfort, and friction whilst maximising independence, self-respect, and dignity.

Assemble the appropriate manual handling equipment and personnel, and help the client into the desired position. Then ensure that the client is comfortable before you return the client's furniture and equipment to their usual places.

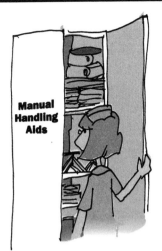

Manual Handling Aids

Safely store away the manual handling equipment. Record in the client's care record when you find a method of moving/handling that is acceptable to all. Also record any problems you encountered in manual handling and/or if you noticed any changes in the client's health or abilities.

Exercise 5.18 🖉

Remember the following rules:

- Always use manual handling aids, when they are available and appropriate for the task in hand. Make sure that the aids are in good working order.

- The task must be designed so that it avoids stooping and/or twisting with a load.

- Pushing and pulling are preferred to lifting a load (although not totally risk-free).

- Take into account the possibility that the load might move suddenly (e.g., the client becomes aggressive or faints).

- Use handling aids, rather than grasp a client under the armpits.

- Beware of space constraints. Although some furniture can be moved out of the way, narrow toilets, wheelchairs, etc., always make manual handling more difficult. If unsure, use a hoist.

- Make sure you are dressed appropriately for manual handling (i.e., loose fitting clothing and flat heeled shoes).

- Adaptations to planned manual handling tasks may need to be used if activities in addition to manual handling have to be undertaken at the same time (e.g., inserting a bedpan, adjusting clothing, guarding clinical equipment such as catheters and intravenous infusions).

- The usual way to coordinate a manual handling task is to say, "1-2-3-move/slide." Some care workers commence the move on "3" and some on "move/slide." Therefore, it is suggested the words "ready-brace-push/slide/pull/stand" should be used.

- Evaluate each manual handling operation. If any changes or adaptations are required, make sure that these are well documented.

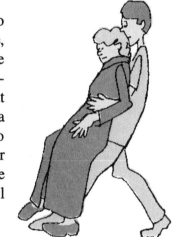

- If a client appears to be falling at any time, do not try to catch the person. Simply provide support so that he or she falls in a controlled fashion to the floor, bed, or chair, minimising the risk of injuries to all concerned.

- If you find a client on the floor, make him or her as comfortable as possible, but do not attempt to move the person until properly assessed for injuries. Always use a hoist to get a client up from the floor, unless he or she can get him/herself up, or unless the position puts the client in further danger.

- Do not utilise personnel for manual handling unless they have been appropriately trained for the moves and equipment that are to be used, and you are sure that they are physically fit enough for the task.

- If a safe manual handling solution cannot be found, the client should remain in bed until appropriate equipment can be obtained.

- If the client's preferences conflict with safe practice, inform the person-in-charge.

- Any long-term environmental constraints to manual handling (e.g., steps, uneven floor, narrow doorway) should be reported so that the environment can be speedily adapted for the needs of the client(s).

Exercise 5.19 ✎

The experience of being moved physically by others can be unpleasant and frightening, especially if no prior explanation or warning has been given by the care workers to the client. Following are the aims of utilising manual handling equipment:

- Help clients to achieve more independence.

- Provide a safe way of moving or transferring a client from one place to another.

- Achieve physical comfort whilst maintaining the dignity of clients.

- Minimise the potential hazards of manual handling.

Manual Handling Aids

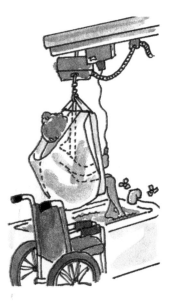

There are at least 60 different types of hoists and 150 manual handling aids available for care settings. Not all care environments provide the manual handling aids that care workers need nor the training to use them. The following examples of manual handling aids improve the care worker's manual handling techniques, while allowing the client more independence.

Hoists can be attached to an overhead track or hung from a mobile stand. The most popular is the hand or battery-operated, mobile hoist that enables a non-weight bearing individual to be transferred from one area to another. The hoists can usually be adapted for a number of lifting tasks, including the use of fixed chairs and slings.

A **transfer belt** fits around a client's waist and has handles. This enables the carer to push, pull, assist, or guide a client without having to bend into a dangerous position or put his or her arms around the client. 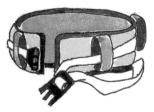 The belt is usually adjustable so that it can fit a variety of people, and it will often include looped hand holds. The belt should not be used for lifting clients. Remember that narrow belts that are unpadded can dig into a client's waist.

A **sliding board** is either a one-piece transfer board which has one low friction surface and a non-smooth surface that 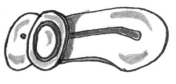 won't slip, or a board that has a sliding section where the friction occurs between the board and the sliding section. A sliding board is simply used to bridge a gap (e.g., between wheelchair and bed) so that the client can slide along the board. The boards come in different sizes, widths, lengths, and curves. They are cheap and portable. The transfer is usually easier if the two surfaces are level and the client has good sitting balance.

Turning discs are usually made of two discs that rotate against each other. There are two main types—the moulded plastic and the flexible fabric. 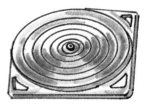 A turning disc can be used, for example, by a person who has just transferred from a wheelchair to a car seat. The device enables the person to swing the feet inside the car.

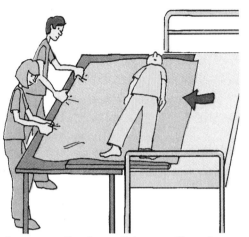

A **supine transfer board** is usually a large, solid board that has one slippery surface to allow the transfer of a supine (laid on back) patient from one level surface to another (e.g., from trolley to bed). It can be used in conjunction with a sliding sheet. The board can be easily stored, and some versions have hand holds or handles built in to the device.

Sliding sheets are available in many forms, including cushioned varieties. They are useful for clients who have difficulty in moving or positioning themselves in bed or who can be safely transferred onto a level surface without the aid of a hoist.

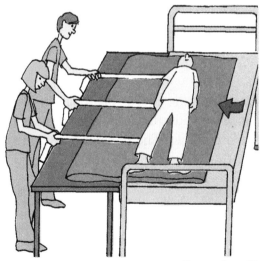

Instead of manually lifting the client, the client is pulled or slid up or across the bed by one or two care workers. Most sliding sheets are tubular in design, with a slippery nylon inner surface and a non-slip outer surface. Some versions have hand holds sewn into the fabric that can be grasped by care workers.

Sliding sheets are especially useful for sliding under clients who have fallen into tight spaces (e.g., a toilet floor) and need to be moved to where a hoist can be used. Preferably, all clients should have their own sliding sheets.

For clients who tend to slide down the bed, in conjunction with a slightly tilted bed, the client can be left on a one way slide sheet. The sheet slides easily in one direction, but prevents sliding in the opposite direction.

A **bed ladder** has solid rungs and rope sides. It is usually attached to the foot of a bed. It is an inexpensive device that allows a client who has good arm strength to grab hold of the lower rungs and gradually climb up the ladder using the hands, until a sitting position is reached.

A **monkey pole** is a swinging bar that hangs over the bed from a metal frame. The client grasps the bar with both hands. This enables the client to lift his or her bottom clear of the bed to relieve pressure, to 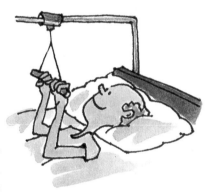 move or turn in bed, to enable a carer to insert a sliding sheet, and/or to strengthen the client's arm muscles. It cannot be used to help a client move up the bed.

Handling slings are positioned under the client's thighs, buttocks, or hips, so that the carer does not have to lean too far forward to achieve a good grip (e.g., when sliding a client up the bed).

Hand blocks are provided for clients who can support their upper bodies, lean forward a little, and have good hand and arm strength. They are placed at either side of a client who is sat in bed so that the client can lift his or her bottom clear of the bed, relieve pressure on the bottom, or move or slide him/herself up the bed.

Exercise 5.20 🖉

As care workers utilise the manual handling aids, they become more proficient in their use. However, even when hoists are being used, there is usually still the need to pull and push the hoist around.

One of the great challenges for care workers is to undertake the manual handling of a confused and/or frightened client. Allow the client to feel calm and safe so that he or she is willing to cooperate and/or help. Utilise a confident tone of voice and a smile. Do not be afraid to leave the client alone for a while to allow time to calm down.

Beds

In relation to caring for clients on beds, you should ask yourself three questions. **First, is the client on the correct type of bed?** In their own homes, clients are cared for on their own beds. In care facilities, many clients are still provided with King's Fund beds. These beds are only considered suitable for clients who have few mobility problems. This applies to few patients admitted to hospitals nowadays.

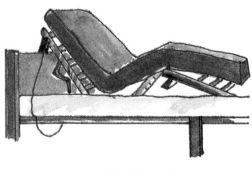

Profiling Bed

The best option is a four-section profiling bed. The bed enables a client to be sat up or laid down in bed without any need for manual handling. In addition, the client can move him/herself, without having to call for help from a carer. Heavy duty and specialist beds are available for very large clients and clients who have specialist health problems (e.g., quadriplegia).

Second, is the client on the correct type of mattress? All clients who are at risk of developing pressure sores should be cared for on one of the types of mattresses that reduce pressure to the "at-risk" areas of the body. The investment in a pressure-relieving mattress more than outweighs the costs of the extra care needed for someone who develops a pressure sore and the misery and discomfort the pressure sore causes.

Third, does the bed allow the use of the manual handling devices that are needed for this client? One problem that can occur here is when the base of the bed prevents the use of a mobile hoist.

Exercise 5.21

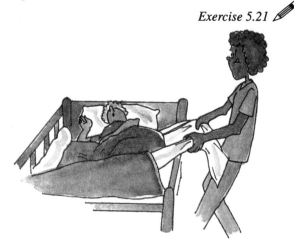

Common Manual Handling Situations

Turning the client in bed is usually referred to as *log rolling*. The manoeuvre is used for a number of reasons (e.g., changing bed linen, inserting hoist slings and slide sheets, as well as turning a client in bed in order to prevent pressure sores, and to aid the drainage of secretions from the lungs). A client will be turned a full 90 degrees for the changing of sheets, but may only be turned/tilted approximately 30 degrees (less than a full turn) for the purpose of trying to relieve the pressure areas.

The best way to turn a client in bed is to use a cushioned sliding sheet which can be left in place, in readiness for the next log roll. The sheets are designed to slide from side to side and allow a client to be turned in bed using minimum effort.

Follow this procedure for turning a client in bed:

1. The bed is raised or lowered to the care worker's waist level.

2. A sliding sheet should be positioned under the client with the open ends of the sheet facing the top and bottom of the bed.

3. The client's head is turned to face the direction of the move.

4. The arm, on the side of the body on which the client is to be rolled, should be bent at the elbow and placed so that it does not end up under the body after the roll.

5. The other arm should be placed across the client's chest.

6. The leg, which will be on top when the client has been rolled onto his or her side, should be slightly bent and pulled forward.

7. Either roll the client towards you, using the shoulder and knee as levers; or pull on the sliding sheet to roll the client, ensuring that there is someone on the opposite side of the bed or that a padded bed side is left up so that the client cannot fall out of bed. Lower the bed side once the procedure has been completed.

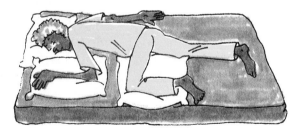

8. Maintain the client's position by the use of pillows behind the client's back and/or between the legs and/or against the chest.

9. Protect the client's skin by ensuring there are no creases in the pillows.

Heavier clients will require two or more carers for the log roll. Additional carers may also be required if the clients are uncooperative or are attached to medical equipment (e.g., urinary catheter, intravenous infusion).

Exercise 5.22 🖎

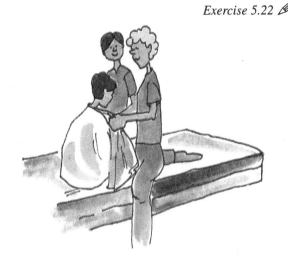

Sitting a client forward in bed is often done by asking the client to bend forward from a supine position. A profiling bed will sit a client up for you automatically. Where possible, always allow a client to sit him/herself up (e.g., by using a bed ladder).

Sitting forward can be very difficult for clients who are frail, confused, unwell, or who have abdominal injuries or wounds. The upper part of the body can be very heavy. You can estimate that, in a paralysed or uncooperative client, you may be exposed to lifting up to a third of the client's body weight. This is obviously unacceptable, and the following techniques are provided only for clients who can help when they are being sat forward in bed.

1. The bed is adjusted to a fairly low position.

2. The care workers stand on either side of the bed and face the client. Each places the inside knee and foot on the bed at the level of the client's hip.

3. The care workers use an elbow to elbow grip with the client's arms.

4. The outside arm of each care worker is then free (e.g., to plump up the client's pillows).

An alternative procedure is to place a draw sheet or folded sheet between the client and the bed, stretching it from hip to shoulder. The care workers kneel on the bed as in the other procedure. The sheet can then be grasped by the care workers and the client can be pulled towards them using the sheet instead of the elbow to elbow grip.

Exercise 5.23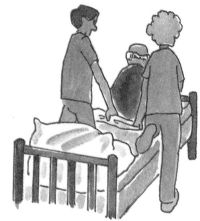

Moving a Seated Client Up or Down the Bed

When in a profiling bed, a client should not need to be moved up or down the bed. If the client has slipped down the bed, the bed can be adjusted into a semi-chair shape, and the client automatically slides back into position.

If a client can help in moving him/herself up the bed, rock the client from side to side onto a fabric slide. The client can then be encouraged to slide up the bed by pushing with the legs and/or by the use of bed blocks. When necessary, additional help can be provided by the care worker. The client bends his or her legs, and the care worker holds the feet in place so that when the client straightens the legs, he or she moves up the bed.

The method outlined here is for clients who can support themselves when sat up in bed. It should *not* be used for people who cannot sit up unsupported; who are confused; who have injuries to their shoulders, chests, or back; or who have little or no control of their heads and necks.

1. The height of the bed is set at waist level. When there are two people of different heights, the waist height of the shorter one dictates the height of the bed.

2. The sliding sheet is positioned underneath the client using a log rolling technique. The open ends of the sheet should be facing the sides of the bed.

3. The bed height is then re-set at just above knee level.

4. The client is helped into a sitting position, with both care workers facing the same way as the client.

5. The inside knee and foot of each care worker is placed on the bed next to the client at the level of his or her buttocks. The outside foot remains on the floor, close to the bed and parallel to the inside knee. The knee of the outside leg is slightly bent.

6. The care worker's inside hand takes hold of the handling sling, whilst the outside hand gently grasps the hand of the client to provide balance and support.

7. One of the care workers takes the lead in commencing the move by saying, e.g., "Ready, brace, slide." The two care workers then sit back onto their heels whilst holding onto the slide, moving the client into the required position.

8. If the client has not moved up the bed enough, the care workers reposition themselves and repeat the move.

Moving On/Off the Bed in a Supine Position

This move is often used for unconscious clients, and it most commonly occurs between the bed and a trolley and between a trolley and an operating table. Despite what you see on the television, there is no safe way to lift a supine client from one flat surface to another. Even poles and canvas are now thought to be unsafe for the transfer.

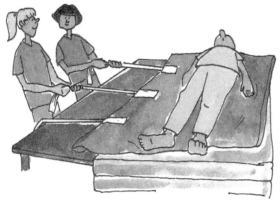

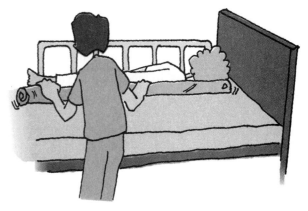

The easiest and safest way is to use a hard or soft sliding device. The devices are all used in a similar fashion.

1. Half roll the client away from the direction of travel using a log rolling technique, and insert the slide.

2. Then roll the client back onto the slide.

3. Push or pull the client across to the other surface.

4. Remove the slide. This can usually be removed without having to move the client again.

Exercise 5.24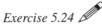

Changing bed linen with the client in the bed is only carried out when a client is on full bed rest and is not allowed to get out of bed. The basic method is to adapt the log rolling technique.

1. The client is rolled onto his or her side, and the soiled bed linen is tightly rolled up behind the client. If necessary, the bed and mattress can be cleaned, disinfected, and dried at this point. The client can also be cleansed and have the pressure areas checked.

2. A clean sheet is then put in place where the soiled bed linen has been removed, and the excess is rolled up tightly behind the client, next to the soiled linen. If necessary, an incontinence pad can be used to create a barrier between the clean and soiled linen to prevent the clean linen from becoming soiled.

3. The client can then be rolled back over both sets of bed linen, onto his or her other side.

4. The soiled bed linen is now removed and disposed of, and the clean sheet can be pulled out and spread over the whole mattress. If necessary, the client's soiled clothing can be removed and replaced.

5. The client should not be exposed more than necessary during the procedure to prevent chilling and minimise embarrassment.

Toileting

In bed: The insertion of a bedpan is easy if the supine client can bridge (raise the buttocks off the bed). A monkey pole can be useful here. The bedpan is simply slipped under the client without any need for manual handling. If not, the client is rolled onto the side, the bedpan is put in position, and he or she is rolled onto the bedpan. If the client is very heavy, a hoist needs to be used.

Where feasible, the client can then be sat up on the bedpan. It is not uncommon for a person to be unsteady or feel unsafe whilst perched on the bedpan. If necessary, the care worker can support the client when using the bedpan, but most clients prefer privacy. Therefore, when possible, it is better to ensure that the client has bed sides or hand blocks for support.

If a client simply wants to pass urine, it is usually better to use a male or female urinal, as appropriate.

Sometimes a heavy, community-based client can suddenly become dependent and unable to move him/herself. Until a full assessment can be undertaken and a hoist provided, it may be necessary to temporarily catheterise the client.

At the toilet: When a client cannot be safely transferred to the toilet inside a narrow toilet cubicle, it is appropriate to transfer the client to a mobile sanichair outside the cubicle where there is more room. The client can then be pushed over the toilet whilst sat on the sanichair. In this case, the external door to the toilet area will need to be locked so that the client can have privacy for the process.

A sanichair should have castors and a braking mechanism on all four legs. It should also have footrests which can be moved to one side when a client is getting on or off the sanichair.

An individual care worker should not be expected to carry out other tasks whilst supporting a client who is getting up or sitting down on a toilet or sanichair. If the client needs wiping, or if clothing needs to be adjusted, this should be done by another care worker.

If a client is finding mobilisation difficult, it is best to avoid the stress of attempting to get to the toilet in time, as this may lead to a fall. It is better to walk a client back from the toilet, rather than to the toilet. Take the client to the toilet on a wheelchair, and let him or her walk back.

Exercise 5.25

Washing and Bathing

Washing and bathing clients can be hard work for care workers. There are a number of ways that a dependent client can maintain personal hygiene:

- Having a strip wash
- Being given a bed bath
- Having a bath, if appropriate bathing aids are available
- Having a shower whilst seated

These choices should enable you to help a client meet his/her personal hygiene needs whilst maintaining privacy and comfort. Allow the client to be as independent as possible within the bounds of safety.

Care workers should always use a comfortable working posture. Never, under any circumstances, lift a client into or out of the bath. Whenever possible, use non-slip bath aids for sitting or standing. Allow clients who can use a bath to enter from a sitting position, rather than by stepping over the bath side with the accompanying risk of the client slipping or losing balance.

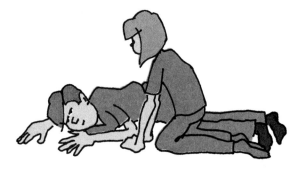

Clients Who Have Collapsed on the Floor

Whether a client has just collapsed or you have simply found a client on the floor, you should first assess the client to see if he or she has suffered a respiratory or cardiac arrest. Then check for injuries, and try and find out why the person collapsed.

Leave the client where he or she is, as long as the person is in no danger, until the person has received treatment or regains consciousness. The only reasons you would attempt to move the client immediately are:

- When you are in water and the client may drown
- When there is danger from a fire, smoke, or fumes
- When there is an obvious physical danger (e.g., from a bomb, a bullet, an aggressive person, falling masonry)

Never try to manually lift a client from the floor. There is a very great risk of injury to the care worker. If the client cannot get him/herself up from the floor, you should use a hoist to move the person. If necessary, slide the person out of a tight space on a sliding sheet first.

Occasionally you will encounter a client who throws him/herself out of bed or who purposely injures oneself against the bed frame. You may have to provide one-to-one care to prevent the client from injuring him/herself. If the human resources are not available, you will have to care for the client on the floor (on a mattress). The client will then have to be lifted by a hoist onto a bed every time you want to provide care. Do not try to provide care at floor level because this will result in you having to use a "risky" posture.

Exercise 5.26 🖉

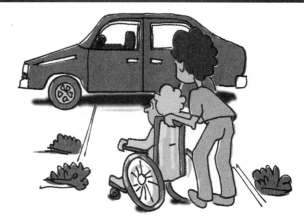

Getting In and Out of a Car

Clients who can stand present few problems when getting in and out of a car. The wheelchair is positioned close to the car so that the person can either slide across, or stand up and lower him/herself into the car seat, before swivelling to get the feet and legs into the car.

When transferring a person with mobility problems into a car, note that a two-door car usually has more

space for the transfer than a four-door car. Never try to transfer a person into the rear seat of a two-door car.

The car should be parked so that the car seat and the wheelchair are on the same level. The footplates of the wheelchair need to be pushed back, and the person's feet are placed on the edge of the car's door frame. The person's bottom should be at the same level as the car seat. The inside armrest of the wheelchair is removed to allow the transfer across to the car seat.

If the person leans away from the car, a transfer board can be placed under him or her to span the gap between wheelchair and car seat. The person then leans slightly forward and slides or shuffles across onto the car seat. The legs should follow and fall into place in front of the car seat. When required, a soft turning disc or a plastic carrier bag can be used to help the person turn after he or she is sitting in the car seat.

Exercise 5.27 🖉

Part 3: Exercising and Improving Mobility (Z6)

Enable others to be as independent as possible in their movements.

Most people enjoy a sense of freedom and well-being that can be achieved by being active and mobile. These positive feelings are denied many clients due to illness and disability. When mobility is restricted for a short period of time, the care staff should support and encourage the client as mobility returns.

Exercise 5.28 🖉

Some clients may have to accustom themselves to long-term restrictions on mobility. This does not mean that they cannot exercise. The emphasis is placed on enabling clients to be as independent as possible and on encouraging them to undertake exercises that improve, maintain, or reduce deterioration in their current level of mobility.

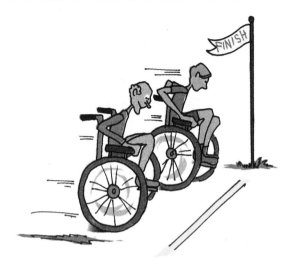

For many people, the word "exercise" conjures up images of jogging, aerobics, and football. The Special Olympics, for people who have mental and physical disabilities, is proof that even very disabled individuals can take up sporting activities. For some clients, this type of exercise may be inappropriate, or even impossible. However, planned and controlled exercise can form an important component of their plan of care.

There are natural opportunities that occur during the day that can provide useful forms of exercise. When you have analysed the exercise that you get at home and elsewhere, you may find opportunities for some of your clients to take more active roles in everyday household activities that will enable them to have some exercise.

Exercise 5.29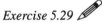

When a client chooses not to move, or moves as little as possible, this in itself can cause a number of health problems (e.g., pressure sores, constipation, urine infections).

Increased fitness and flexibility are important benefits of exercise. Additional benefits include the following:

- Increased sense of inner well-being and improved self-esteem
- Improved appearance by maintaining weight and/or staying slim
- Improved personal health
- Increased energy levels
- Reduced feelings of stress and anxiety, and improvements in the quality of sleep

The main physical benefits of exercise are in the three "Ss"—stamina, strength, and suppleness.

Stamina allows you to undertake normal, everyday activities without feeling tired or getting out of breath and enables your heart and lungs to work harder for longer. Stamina is achieved by participation in activities such as tennis, swimming, and football.

Strength is linked to being able to use your muscles and joints to pull, push, and lift yourself and other objects during activities such as weight training and mountain biking.

Suppleness is the flexibility to be able to bend, stretch, twist, and turn through the full range of movements which can be achieved in yoga and gymnastics. Swimming is often regarded as the best all round exercise because the water counteracts the effects of gravity and there is no impact that can injure joints.

Exercise can be damaging if it is carried out in the wrong way. Damage is usually related to forgetting to stretch and not warming up before exercising, too much exercise for the levels of stamina that are available, and trying to force aching bodies and limbs to be flexible before they are ready to do so.

Exercise 5.30

Active and Passive Exercises

Assisting clients with active and passive exercises is usually the joint responsibility of the physiotherapist and the care worker. The exercises are active when they are performed by the client, and they are passive when performed by the care worker on behalf of the client. They are usually carried out following an anaesthetic and surgery, during periods of unconsciousness, and during periods of reduced mobility (short-term during illness, long-term when a client has a disability).

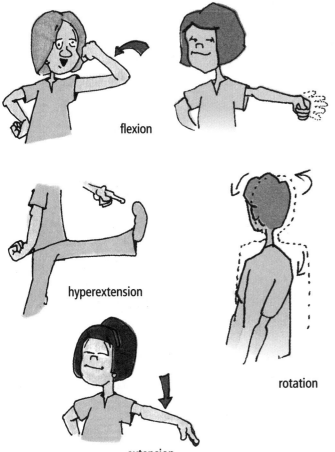

flexion

hyperextension

rotation

extension

There are a number of benefits of active and passive exercises. For example, they increase the client's depth and rate of respiration. This can help reduce the chances of developing a chest infection during periods of reduced mobility. Also, regular exercising for a client who is on enforced bedrest promotes the circulation of the blood and helps to prevent deep vein thrombosis which can result in a pulmonary embolism and death.

Exercises help to maintain muscle tone when there is reduced mobility so that the client can resume normal mobility with minimum joint stiffness or muscle weakness. Exercising a paralysed limb helps to prevent joint stiffness, muscle contracture (permanent shortening of the muscles), and muscle atrophy (wasting away of muscle tissue).

You will need to know the full range of movements that each joint should be put through. If you are not sure about the range of movements for a specific joint, locate the same joint on your own body/limb, and see for yourself the extent of movement through which the joint can be moved. Nearly all joints can be flexed and extended. Some joints can be rotated, and some can be hyperextended.

Exercise 5.31 🖉

Follow these guidelines for active and passive exercises:

1. Wash your hands.

2. Explain what you are going to do so that you can get the client's informed consent and cooperation. If necessary, provide an explanation as to why the exercises are required, and outline the plan of care for the client.

3. Ensure that the client is dressed appropriately and is warm enough to take part in the exercises.

4. If there is not enough room to safely undertake the exercises, with the client's permission, make room for yourself and the client. Where appropriate, ensure privacy throughout the activity.

5. For active exercise, the client will need to warm up so the limbs and muscles will loosen up to get the body ready for exertion.

6. Help the client into a comfortable position for the exercises. The position may have to be changed for different exercises. For passive exercises, the muscles and joints that are not being exercised should be positioned comfortably and/or supported so that injuries do not occur.

7. Whether exercises are active or passive, you will tend to follow the same pattern of exercises. The whole of the spine and trunk are put through the normal range of movements. Each limb is taken separately, and all the joints in the limb are put through the full range of movements.

8. The joint should be supported and moved gently, smoothly, and slowly through the normal range of movements for the client three to five times.

9. Provide feedback and encouragement to a client who is doing his or her own exercises or helping with the exercises. Where appropriate, teach the client to undertake the exercises by him/herself.

10. Never force a joint or muscle through any range of movements as this could cause an injury and further reduce mobility.

11. If a joint is hot, red, and swollen, do not exercise it.

12. Observe the client's face for signs of discomfort or pain. If pain occurs, stop the exercises. Try to make sure that the client is not in pain or in too much discomfort during the exercises. Report any problems to the person-in-charge.

13. If the client is undertaking active exercises, include a "cooling down" period towards the end of the session to enable the client to gently slow down the exercises and cool off.

14. Observe the client throughout the activity so that you can report back on any problems encountered and improvements or deterioration in the client's mobility that you have noticed during the exercises.

15. Make sure the client is comfortable. If necessary, restore the client's physical environment back to its original condition.

16. Wash your hands.

17. If required, make a record that the passive/active movements have been undertaken and any other relevant facts that need to be reported. You may be required to monitor the after effects of the exercises on the client.

Where appropriate, plan exercises into the clients' normal daily activities. For example, clients who can clean their own teeth should, at the same time, be able to put their shoulders, arms, wrists, and fingers through the whole range of movements required for exercise purposes.

Exercise 5.32 🖉

Maintaining Client Mobility

A client may lose mobility unnecessarily. The client may be frightened to move for fear of falling. Perhaps the client is overweight or spends too much time in bed due to a lack of help and support to get up. Sometimes a client learns to become dependent on others who do things for him or her.

You cannot force a client to become more mobile. Therefore, before care is planned, you need to know whether the client wants to be more mobile. You also need to know whether the resources are available in your area of care to take the action that is required to improve the client's mobility.

Exercise 5.33 🖉

Guidelines on the manual handling of clients are provided in Part 2 of this module.

When standing a client up, use precautions.

- Do not lift a client manually to a standing position.

- Do not encourage a client to move to a standing position unless you are reasonably sure the client can take his or her own weight with minimal support and assistance.

- When a client is to stand from a sitting position, make sure he or she is in an appropriate chair (i.e., the chair should not be too soft, too low, or too deep).

- Check whether the client uses a walking stick or walking frame for balance and support.

- Ensure there is enough room for the client and for you to provide support.

- Ensure the client's clothing and shoes are appropriate for the task.

- Provide as little support as is needed so that the client can be as independent as possible.

Follow this procedure for standing a client up:

1. If the client needs support whilst standing, ensure that he or she wears a handling belt.

2. Ask the client to shuffle the hips forward so that he or she is sat forward on the seat.

3. Ask the client to lean forward with the nose over the toes.

4. Ensure that the feet are positioned so that one knee is at a right angle with the foot flat on the floor, and the other foot is positioned to the side slightly behind the first foot.

5. If necessary, rock the client back and forwards a couple of times, prior to standing, in order to gain the momentum necessary to stand.

6. Ask the client to straighten the legs whilst using the arms of the chair for support, and then encourage the client to stand erect and look straight ahead.

7. On standing, once the client feels balanced, he or she can then grasp the walking stick or walking frame before moving away.

8. Make sure that there are enough carers present to provide the support that the client needs. If, at any point, the client appears to be losing his or her balance or starts to fall, do not try to catch the person, just lower the person as gently as possible back into the chair.

If a client has previously fallen, you must take extra care. Do not allow yourself to be used as a prop.

Exercise 5.34 🖉

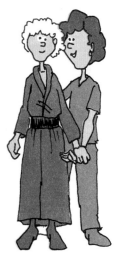

When **helping a client to walk**, the care worker is usually positioned at the side of the client. Although you are providing support at waist height, the load must be taken on one side, leading to the spine being unbalanced. If a client starts to fall or faint, you will have to twist to provide support, and this is very dangerous. If you are not well matched with the client in terms of height, you should be especially careful. Preferably, the client should wear a handling belt.

If there is only one care worker available, he or she should stand on the client's weak side, holding the client's right hand in his or her right hand (or vice versa). The client's arm should be straight so that the client can press down with the palm on the care worker's palm (thumbs interlocking) to gain support.

Where necessary, the client can be followed around by another care worker pushing a wheelchair in case the client becomes tired and needs to sit down quickly. If the client starts to fall, release the client's hand, move behind the client, and take one step back so that you can provide some support as the client slides to the floor.

Exercise 5.35 🖉

Mobility Aids

Mobility aids are assistive devices that enable clients—physically and psychologically—to regain the highest level of mobility possible. It is your responsibility to make sure that the mobility aids are in good repair and are used correctly. If you notice any defects or problems with a mobility aid, report them promptly so that repairs can be quickly carried out and accidents prevented.

Provide clients with relevant information on the use and maintenance of their mobility aids. Explain in a manner and at a pace and level they can understand, especially in terms of safety when negotiating different types of floor surface (e.g., uneven, sloping, stairs). When a mobility aid is being used, always ensure that the immediate area is cleared of potential hazards.

Make sure that you know the correct way a mobility aid should be used before helping someone else to use it. If required, demonstrate the use of the mobility aid. Some clients may need quite a lot of encouragement before they feel confident to use the mobility aid independently. Provide the client with the necessary support, encouragement, and feedback so that mobility appliances are used correctly and safely. Always keep the mobility aid within easy reach for the client.

Mark the client's name on the mobility aid in an inconspicuous place for identification purposes. This includes marking the removable parts of wheelchairs. Encourage clients to care for and clean their own mobility aids, if they are able, before and after use.

If a mobility device appears to be no longer appropriate for use by a client, seek advice from an experienced colleague (e.g., physiotherapist). Any defective or broken mobility aid should be labelled and taken out of circulation for repair or disposal. Check for any physical problems related to using the mobility aid (e.g., pinching, swelling, rubbing, sore spots).

Exercise 5.36

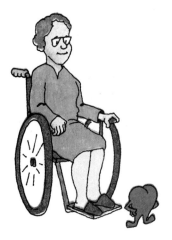

When using a **wheelchair**, ensure that the client is properly positioned for comfort and safety. Wheelchairs are equipped with a variety of options including removable armrests, footrests, seat cushions, and devices to ensure that the client is correctly positioned in the wheelchair.

All of these components are potential causes of injury or discomfort to a client. If the wheelchair is used by more than one person, ensure that it is appropriately adjusted for each new person who has to use it.

To maintain wheelchairs, check for loose, worn, or missing parts, and check the brakes regularly. Oil moving metal components of the wheelchair regularly, and keep the chair clean.

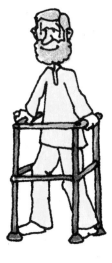

Walking frames are usually prescribed by doctors or physiotherapists. The most common type of walking frame is the Zimmer frame. The type of Zimmer frame that is used depends on the client's abilities, needs, and preferences. A *standard* Zimmer frame is rigid with four legs. It is used for balance. A *gliding* Zimmer frame is similar to the standard Zimmer frame except that there are wheels on the front legs so that it can be pushed, rather than having to be picked up. Alternatively, a *reciprocal* walker has a hinged frame that moves forward one side at a time.

Be aware that clients can fall when using walkers. Take special care with obstacles that are in the path as some walking frames need quite a lot of space to be used safely.

Make sure that the frame is the correct size for the person who is using it. The majority of walking frames can be adjusted for height. When you re-adjust the height, ensure that the positioning buttons are correctly positioned so that the walker does not suddenly collapse under the client's weight.

To maintain walking frames, check for loose screws and worn tips. Always ensure that mobility aids are safe *before* clients use them.

Canes are used by clients to provide balance and to partially support the client's weight on one side of the body. For balance, the cane is usually used on the client's strong side. For supporting weight, it is usually used on the client's weak side. Care should be taken when the client is learning to use the cane to ensure that he or she does not fall.

To maintain canes, check the tips for worn or missing rubber/plastic cups. Also, check canes for cracks or loose screws.

Exercise 5.37 ✎

Crutches are placed under the client's armpits to take all or most of the weight off one foot or leg. The client should be checked regularly to prevent sore armpits. Crutches can take some getting used to. Take great care when the client is learning to use the crutches to ensure that he or she does not fall.

To maintain crutches, check the tips for worn or missing rubber/plastic cups, and check for cracks or loose screws. Also, check the padding for wear.

Exercise 5.38 ✎

Part 4: Providing Pressure Area Care (Z7.3)

Minimise the effects of pressure on skin.

The skin is the body's largest organ. It is easily damaged. The skin of people who are ill or old is especially vulnerable. Lying or sitting in one position for too long causes pressure over bony prominences. Pressure affects the blood supply to the skin and underlying tissues. If an area of skin does not receive an adequate blood supply, it becomes damaged and may die.

Exercise 5.39 ✎

Preventing problems is much easier than healing damaged skin. The people who are most at risk from pressure sores are those who:

- Are immobile and inactive
- Are incontinent
- Are unconscious
- Are overweight or underweight
- Have an infection or circulatory disease
- Have poor personal hygiene

Pressure Sores

The terms *pressure sore* and *decubitus ulcer* are used to describe an area of damage to the skin or underlying tissue caused by direct pressure or shearing forces. Pressure sores tend to occur over the body's bony prominences (noted in the illustration below).

Pressure sores develop in four stages:

1. A pink or red area on the skin does not disappear within 15 minutes after the pressure has been relieved.

2. The skin is cracked, blistered, or broken and the surrounding area is red.

3. The skin breaks down, and the subcutaneous tissue is exposed.

4. The sore penetrates to the muscle or bone, and there may be infection and drainage of fluid.

Exercise 5.40 ✎

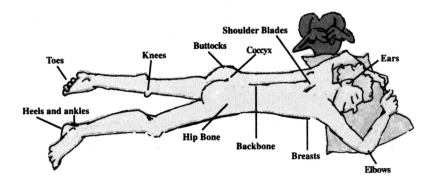

To prevent pressure sores, follow these general guidelines:

Relieve pressure: Rotate an immobile client's position every two hours. Use appropriate pressure-relieving devices to redistribute the pressure and support pillows to maintain position.

Prevent friction and shearing: Never rub the skin vigorously (that includes rubbing with soap and water and/or oil). Avoid dragging a person in bed as this can shear the skin, and avoid wrinkles in sheets and clothing on which a person is sat or laid.

Control moisture: Keep the clients clean and dry (especially if they are incontinent or perspiring heavily).

Prevent skin trauma: Keep your nails short so that you do not accidentally scratch someone. Do not wear jewelry or badges that could damage a client's skin.

Exercise 5.41 🖉

Make sure that all of the clients in your care have been assessed using a recognised pressure area assessment tool (e.g., Norton or Waterlow), that has been ratified by your employing organisation. When there is a change in a client's condition, the client should be reassessed.

Do not rub any areas at risk of developing pressure sores as this may cause damage or degeneration of the skin. Only wash the areas of the body at risk if the client has been incontinent or has been sweating profusely. Ensure that all the soap is rinsed off and that the area is patted, rather than rubbed, dry. If the skin is dry, a moisturiser may be used. Ask clients about their preferences, and only use a barrier cream when needed.

Educate and encourage the client to regularly change position. Provide help, when needed. This can be incorporated into a physiotherapy, occupational therapy, and/or mobility programme, and other activities of daily living. If the client cannot regularly examine the pressure areas, do it for him or her.

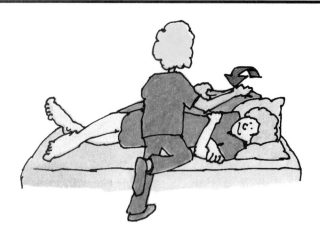

If necessary, turn the client at least every two hours, recording the client's position on the relevant chart each time he or she has been turned. The majority of clients should be encouraged to sit up in chairs or in bed. Where possible, use a bean bag to help with positioning in bed, rather than the bed's backrest. The periods of time that a client can be left sat up in a chair may need to be reduced if sacral or pelvic sores start to develop.

Where possible, clients should be involved in their own care planning to minimise the effects of pressure. Remember to use a level and pace of discussion that is appropriate for each client. Inform clients about the factors that cause pressure sores, and encourage them to be as active as possible. Doing as much as they can for themselves results in the pressure being relieved naturally.

Remember that you are caring for the whole client, not just the pressure areas. Encourage the client to be assertive in providing ongoing feedback on the level of comfort or discomfort, and take the client's preferences into account when providing care.

Whilst positioning and supporting the client in a manner that minimises pressure, you will also need to ensure that other needs are taken into consideration, including comfortable clothing and appropriate positioning.

Dress the client so that the mode of dress is as "normal" as possible (e.g., unless the client is ill, it would be inappropriate to be dressed in pyjamas all the time). Ensure that clothing does not inhibit pressure area care (e.g., by being too tight), and that it does not cause pressure sores (from creases, buttons, zips, and seams).

Position the client so that the client can see as much of the environment as possible and can engage in social activities (e.g., converse with other clients, participate in a game of draughts). The position should allow the person to be as self-caring as possible (e.g., feeding, personal hygiene).

Ensure that the plan of care relating to pressure areas is carried out as specified in the care plan. If you encounter any problems in carrying out the plan of care (e.g., the client's condition changes or other care needs require the care plan to be changed), immediately report this to the person-in-charge.

Exercise 5.42 ✏

Clients who are at a high risk of developing pressure sores should be checked more often (e.g., every time you change a client's position). You need to have an awareness of normal skin colours for different racial groups before you can detect the changes that occur due to developing pressure sores.

Pressure-Relieving Equipment

Because some clients cannot change their positions on a regular basis, a variety of devices have been produced for relieving pressure to specific areas of the body. These can be used to prevent pressure sores from developing or to relieve pressure once a pressure sore has developed. Pressure-relieving equipment should be used, cleaned, maintained, and stored in accordance with the manufacturer's instructions.

Relieve the pressure over those parts of the body that are vulnerable to breaking down into pressure sores. When available, use one or more of the pressure-relieving devices described in the next column. The choice of pressure-relieving device must be specific to meet a client's individual need.

- A **sheepskin** is warm and comfortable under the body, and is particularly good at protecting heels, (although it does not relieve the pressure). A sheepskin will tend to harden and matt after it has been washed several times. It needs changing frequently and is not appropriate for clients who are regularly incontinent.

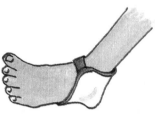

- **Heel and elbow pads** can be made of sheepskin, foam, or silicone. The pads reduce friction and shearing forces to elbows and heels. They can sometimes be difficult to keep in place, and they harden with repeated washing.

- **Pressure-relieving mattresses** include low air loss mattress, alternating pressure mattress, bead mattress, and fibre filled overlay mattress. One of the most commonly used mattresses is the alternating pressure mattress which can be made to fit any bed. It reduces the frequency (but not the need for) regular turning. Despite being prone to break down, the mattresses are comfortable and can be wiped down and disinfected when used for incontinent clients.

- **Special beds** are used when the client is too ill to be moved very much (e.g., spinal injuries units). Here, for example, a rocker bed can be used so that the bed can be tilted to shift the client's position, rather than the client having to be moved on the bed.

Exercise 5.43 ✏

The **treatment of pressure sores** is the same as for any other wound. Care should be focused on relieving the cause (pressure, shearing forces) and minimising the symptoms from any underlying health problems.

Summary

Clients depend on you to help manage their pain and achieve whatever level of comfort is possible. Involve the client in planning care, and be clear about your expected role in minimising pain and discomfort. Pain assessment, therapies, and control are based on each client's individual needs. Help clients meet their needs for adequate rest and sleep in order to promote health and healing.

A major concern is the moving and positioning of clients. Never undertake any manual handling task unless you have received appropriate training. It is important that you use only those manual handling techniques that have been accepted by your employing organisation as safe (for both the clients and those providing care). Ensure that clients who have mobility problems undertake active or passive exercises in order to prevent further health problems from developing. This includes measures to prevent pressure sores.

Check Your Knowledge and Understanding

1. A client has been admitted to your hospital unit for an uncomfortable investigative procedure—a barium enema (opaque dye inserted into the rectum so that the bowel and any abnormalities can be highlighted via X-ray). Six clients have undergone the same procedure, and he is the only one who is complaining of pain. None of the clients have been prescribed any analgesia by a doctor. What would you do?

   a) Ask the client if he has a low pain/discomfort threshold.

   b) Immediately report that the client is in pain to the person-in-charge of the unit so that she can ensure that a speedy pain assessment is carried out by one of the nurses and that the doctor is informed of the situation.

   c) Ask the person-in-charge to provide you with some analgesia for the client.

   d) Point out to the client that he is the only one of the six clients who have undergone the same investigative procedure who is complaining of pain.

2. You are caring for a middle-aged woman in the community who has continuing mild to moderate pain after having an attack of herpes zoster to one side of her face. She has been prescribed an analgesic medication in small tablet form which is effective for relieving the pain, but the woman does not like taking tablets because they tend to get "stuck in her throat." What would you suggest?

   a) Suggest to the client that she might like to try an alternative method of pain relief (e.g., relaxation, distraction) when the pain is mild, saving the analgesic medication for when her face feels very painful.

   b) Remind the client that the analgesic tablets are very effective and, therefore, she should continue to take them, even though she finds them difficult to swallow.

   c) Ask the client if she would like to try to wean herself off the tablets by only taking them when her face is very painful.

   d) Advise the client to visit her doctor to ask if there are any smaller tablets that can be prescribed for her.

3. A rather large client has asked to be moved up the bed. An experienced member of the care staff who comes over to help you states that she does not like all these "new fangled" sliding sheets and devices and refuses to use them. She suggests that you use the Australian (shoulder) lift to move the client up the bed. What would you do?

   a) Go ahead and use the Australian lift because there is nobody else available to help you at the moment.

   b) Insist that the other member of staff helps you to use a slide sheet to move the client.

   c) Slide the person up the bed by yourself.

   d) Gently explain that you would prefer to use the equipment that is provided for this purpose as it is safer for everyone concerned and, therefore, you will wait until someone else is available to help you.

4. A man has been admitted to your care facility after having a minor stroke. He cannot walk and has to be propped up in bed. He needs help with all his self-care needs. He says he would like to have a bath, and he insists that the hoist is not used to get him into and out of the bath. What would you do?

    a) Insist that if the man wants to have a bath, the hoist must be used. Alternatively, he can have a bed bath.

    b) Suggest the man could use the shower instead.

    c) Agree to take the man to the bathroom in his wheelchair and then slide him into and out of the bath from the wheelchair.

    d) Offer the man a strip wash in the communal washroom.

5. One of your clients, an elderly lady who has severe arthritis, has been diagnosed as terminal cancer. She is going to die within the next couple of days. You know that if this lady is not kept mobile, her joints will stiffen up. But, when you go to the lady's bed she insists that she just wants to be left alone with her family to die in peace. What would you do?

    a) Ask the family members who are present at the bedside to leave whilst you carry out active and passive exercises with the client so that her joints do not stiffen up.

    b) Show the family members how to carry out the exercises so that they can do them on your behalf.

    c) Sit down with the client and her family and discuss with them how best you can maintain her comfort over the next couple of days.

    d) Agree to leave the client in peace, as requested.

6. You are asked to care for a man who recently had a stroke that has affected the left side of his body. He has some movement in his left arm and leg but has not been receiving physiotherapy since he left hospital. The man appears to be unable to fully straighten his affected arm and leg. What should you do?

    a) Contact the physiotherapist and wait until the client can be fully assessed before taking any action.

    b) With the client's permission, immediately implement an active exercise regime with special emphasis on his left arm and leg.

    c) Contact the physiotherapist so that the client can be properly assessed. Whilst waiting for the assessment, commence a programme of active and passive exercises on the client's left arm and leg whilst encouraging him to be as independent and self-caring as possible.

    d) Simply accept that the client's left arm and leg are never going to be much use to him. Concentrate on enabling the man to do as much as he can for himself using his right arm and leg.

7. One of your clients has developed a chest infection. Usually he is quite healthy and fully mobile. But, at the moment, he has spent the last two days in bed. He has complained that his bottom is getting sore. When you inspect the area, you notice a small red area of skin around the sacrum. What would you do?

    a) Immediately place the client on an alternating pressure mattress, and commence two-hourly turning.

    b) Place a sheepskin mattress cover under the man. Wash and dry the sacral area thoroughly, and ask him to keep turning himself so that he does not develop a pressure sore.

    c) Undertake a Waterlow pressure area assessment, and then prepare a plan of care to overcome this problem.

    d) Ask the man to lie on his side, rather than remain sat up in bed.

Module 6

Maintaining Hygiene, Nourishment, and Elimination

Help others with their activities of daily living.

Need-to-know words:

- anus
- dehydration
- fluid balance
- halitosis
- menarche
- menopause
- oedema
- oesophagus
- orthosis
- perianal
- prostate gland
- prosthesis
- urethra

Objectives:

- Recognise that people have different standards of personal hygiene and appearance.
- Help others to maintain their appearance and personal hygiene.
- Describe the components of a healthy diet.
- List the different types of diet that are available to clients.
- Monitor a client's fluid balance.
- Help dependent clients to eat and drink.
- Outline the main elimination problems that clients face.
- Describe how to monitor a client's elimination patterns.
- Enable dependent clients to use toilet facilities.
- Outline how to dispose of client body waste.

Module 6 Introduction

Module 6 relates to three units of the level 2 NVQ/SVQ Award in Care:

Unit Z9: **Enable clients to maintain personal hygiene and appearance** is an option group B unit. It consists of two elements of competence:

- Z9.1 Enable clients to maintain their personal cleanliness.

- Z9.2 Support clients in personal grooming and dressing.

Unit Z10: **Enable clients to eat and drink** is an option group B unit. It consists of two elements of competence:

- Z10.1 Help clients to get ready for eating and drinking.

- Z10.2 Help clients to consume food and drink.

Unit Z11: **Enable clients to access and use toilet facilities** is an option group B unit. It consists of three elements of competence:

- Z11.1 Enable clients to use toilet facilities.

- Z11.2 Assist clients to use toilet facilities.

- Z11.3 Collect and dispose of client body waste.

Part 1: Promoting Available Services and Facilities (Z9)

Maintain hygiene and appearance.

Everyone has personal standards of hygiene and appearance. These are shaped by how each person was raised as a child, life experiences, and personal preferences. It is very easy to be critical about the personal hygiene and appearance of other people, especially when their beliefs, lifestyles, and preferred behaviours are different to yours.

Exercise 6.1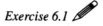

As a care support worker, you may have to help individuals to perform activities linked to personal hygiene and appearance. This can be embarrassing for clients, especially if they are used to doing these activities independently or if the activities are intimate and embarrassing in nature. Therefore, you should be aware that some people find this subject rather difficult to talk about.

Where possible and appropriate, clients should be allowed to make choices as to how they would prefer to maintain their personal hygiene and appearance.

For example, ask them:

- Whether they would prefer baths or showers

- How much of the washing they can do for themselves and how much help they need/want

- How and when they want to carry out the personal hygiene/grooming tasks

- When and how they usually clean their teeth

- How they prefer their nails to look

- What are their preferred toiletries and methods of cleansing

- Who is going to launder their clothes

Personal Hygiene

Hygiene can be described as the practice of providing a level of cleanliness that has a positive effect on health. Personal hygiene is important for a number

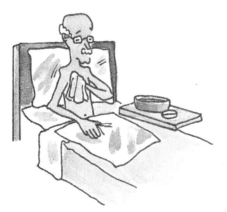

of reasons (e.g., to keep the skin in good condition; to help prevent pressure sores and skin infections from developing; to promote self-esteem, dignity, and a feeling of healthy well-being).

Most people are happy to take on the responsibility for meeting this fundamental need. Always encourage people to meet their own self-hygiene needs where possible.

Exercise 6.2

Unfortunately, there can be problems. People who are very young, very ill, very confused, or very disabled may have trouble maintaining their own hygiene. Also, people who do not have easy access to hygiene resources—soap, towel, running water, toothpaste and toothbrush, etc.—may find it difficult to maintain their personal hygiene. Remember that hygiene and cleanliness are not luxuries, they are basic human rights.

Some people choose lifestyles that can best be described as unhygienic (e.g., people who choose to eat discarded food from litter bins and refuse to wash). Many people have some aspects of their lives that are unhygienic (e.g., forgetting to wash their hands before eating food). You may enjoy washing or the fresh feeling that a bath or shower gives you. For other people, these activities may be a chore, especially if they have disabilities which make the activities difficult to carry out, or if they cause discomfort, or if they do not have easy access to appropriate washing/bathing facilities.

You can set a good example by using high standards of personal hygiene. However, people have their own (different) standards of "hygiene." Therefore, when caring for others, accept their hygiene standards, rather than try to impose your own onto them.

Exercise 6.3

It is appropriate to intervene when people's standards of hygiene are dangerous to themselves or others (e.g., coughing over food that they are preparing for others), or socially unacceptable (e.g., their body odour is making other people feel sick).

In these cases you should try to persuade the person to accept some health education or support in undertaking personal hygiene. The care support worker's role is to try and achieve a "mutually acceptable" level of cleanliness. This can be achieved by a range of measures. Following are examples:

- Arranging to have an open and honest chat about the problem with the person, in private

- Offering support, encouragement, and assistance, as needed

- Being aware that the use of prostheses and orthoses can make it more difficult to maintain personal hygiene

- Offering more bath/shower opportunities

- Arranging to ensure that the client can have privacy whilst seeing to his/her own personal hygiene needs

- Arranging for the client to have better access to clean clothes and toiletries

- Negotiating ways to overcome soreness, pain, or discomfort while maintaining personal hygiene

- Offering the client a single bedroom, rather than a shared bedroom

If the client refuses to change his or her unacceptable personal hygiene habits, seek advice.

Privacy is also a basic human right. For some cultures (e.g., Moslem), modesty is very important and can cause problems when a client cannot manage his or her own personal hygiene and needs to depend on another person for help. Most people feel a sense of embarrassment when another person is required to help them, or undertake for them, some aspect of their personal hygiene that would normally be very private.

In care establishments, there can be common use of care equipment (e.g., bowls, nail scissors). If these are not changed or thoroughly cleansed between clients, there is a serious risk of cross-infection. Where possible, each client should have his or her own toiletries, towel, bowl, etc.

In some care settings, the maintenance of the personal hygiene of clients is viewed by care workers as being a chore to be completed as quickly as possible, especially when there is a shortage of care staff. Maintaining a client's personal hygiene is an essential aspect of care. It provides good opportunities to communicate with the client and assess a client's needs. You are expected to behave in a friendly, caring, and supportive manner.

Avoid, at all costs, appearing indifferent, bored, rushed, or nauseous, even if you really do feel that way. Otherwise you are likely to create feelings of shame, embarrassment, and hostility in the client. Also, if you wear protective clothing, tell the client in an appropriate manner that it is for the client's protection as well as yours.

If you encounter any conflicts between client choice, good hygiene practice, and the client's plan of care, discuss these issues with a more experienced colleague, or report the matter to the person-in-charge.

Exercise 6.4 ✎

Bathing

Bathing provides more than cleanliness. Baths can encourage exercise, stimulate circulation, help prevent pressure sores, and promote relaxation. Baths also provide the opportunity to communicate with a client and spot problems such as skin infections, movement difficulties, etc.

Always encourage and provide opportunities for your clients to wash and bathe themselves, if they are able. Provide a level of privacy that is appropriate to the level of risk in leaving clients alone, and ensure that clients are able to call for help, if required.

Some healthy and mobile clients may need help to wash their feet, backs, and buttocks. This help in maintaining personal hygiene should be provided in a manner which promotes their dignity and minimises discomfort. Many people prefer to get all their personal hygiene and grooming tasks completed in one go. When showering, for example, they may want to wash their hair, clean their teeth, have a shave, etc., whilst they are in the bathroom.

For a **general or tub bath**, use this procedure :

1. Wash your hands.

2. Assemble the equipment—towels, soap or shower gel, wash cloth, clean clothes (if required).

3. Fill the bath half full, running the cold water into the bath first. (It is not uncommon for clients to scald themselves in the bath.)

4. Close any windows and doors, if necessary, for privacy and to ensure that the room temperature is satisfactory for the person.

5. If required, help the person to undress. Make sure that he or she is undressed for the least amount of time necessary before entering the bath. If necessary, the person can put on a bath gown until it is time to enter the bath.

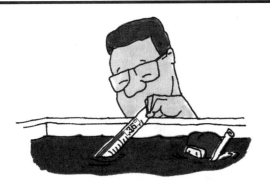

6. Test the water temperature with a bath thermometer before the person enters the bath. The water should be approximately 36 degrees Celsius. If a bath thermometer is not available, test the water temperature with your hand, and ask the person who is having the bath to check that the water temperature is satisfactory.

7. Ensure that there is a non-slip bath mat in the bath.

8. If the person is walking into the bath, ensure that there is a non-slip bath mat (and chair, if necessary) at the side of the bath.

9. If the person cannot get into the bath him/herself, or if there is any danger of the person slipping or falling, do not try and lift or slide the person into the bath. Utilise a hoist to safely lift the person into the bath. (See Module 5, Part 2.)

10. Assist the person, if required, as specified in the plan of care, with washing, rinsing, drying, and dressing.

11. Remove and dispose of all used equipment and waste. Clean the facilities for the next use.

12. Wash your hands.

Exercise 6.5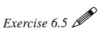

For a **shower**, use this procedure:

1. Wash your hands.

2. Assemble the same equipment as for a tub bath.

3. Where appropriate, use a shower chair for safety so that the person does not have to stand for long periods of time.

4. Close any windows and doors, if necessary, for privacy and to ensure that the room temperature is satisfactory for the person.

5. If required, help the person to undress. Make sure that the person is undressed for the least amount of time necessary before entering the shower. If necessary, the person can put on a bath gown until it is time to enter the shower.

6. Check the water temperature (or ask the client to check the water temperature) before the client goes under the shower.

7. If necessary, assist the person into the shower and onto the shower chair. (See Module 5, Part 2 for safe transfer procedures.)

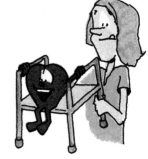

8. Assist, where required according to the plan of care, with washing, rinsing, drying, and re-dressing.

9. Remove and dispose of all used equipment and waste. Clean the facilities for the next use.

10. Wash your hands.

Exercise 6.6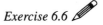

Safety Guidelines for Bathing/Showering

- Use extreme caution to prevent slips and falls.

- Test the water temperature yourself, and then let the client test the water temperature.

- Assist a client in and out of the shower/bath, if required.

- Check the plan of care before leaving a client alone to bathe.

When clients cannot leave their beds to use the bath or shower, they require bed baths. Find out the clients' personal preferences for their hygiene and their self-care abilities before commencing bed baths. The bed bath is an excellent opportunity for communicating with the client and assessing the client's physical condition.

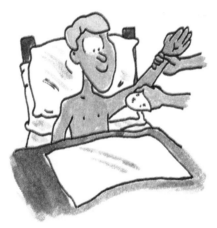

For a **bed bath,** use this procedure:

1. Wash your hands.

2. Collect all necessary equipment at the bedside—clean bed linen, bath towel, laundry skip, towel(s), toiletries, clean night clothes, inco wipes, washbasin, and warm water.

3. Clear the area around the bed. Ensure privacy by pulling curtains or screens, and closing doors. Close all nearby windows to prevent draughts.

4. Allow the client the chance to use a bedpan, commode, or urinal before you commence the bed bath.

5. Cover the client with a bath blanket over the bed clothes, and then pull the bed clothes down to the foot of the bed.

6. Fill the bowl with hot water and commence by washing the hands and face; ask if soap is required. Any additional care of the mouth, eyes, ears, or nose care can be given after the bed bath.

7. Remove the top half of the client's clothing so that the top half of the body can be washed, rinsed, and dried. Take special care with skin folds (e.g., the axillae, under the breasts). Avoid spilling water onto the bed. Apply toiletries where requested, and replace the clothing.

8. Change the water at this point, or at any other point in the bed bath, when the water becomes cool or very soapy.

9. Remove the bottom half of the client's clothing (if necessary), ensuring that only those parts of the body that are being washed/dried are exposed.

10. Wash, rinse, and dry the lower part of the body. Ensure that the genital and anal areas are washed using inco wipes and that the water is changed afterwards.

11. Apply toiletries where requested, and replace the clothing.

12. Change the bottom sheet whilst the client is being turned during the bed bath.

13. Where necessary, assist the client with dental hygiene, and provide help to comb or brush the hair.

14. Pull the bed clothes back up over the client, and remove the bath blanket.

15. Remove and dispose of all used equipment, and wash your hands.

Exercise 6.7 🖉

After bathing, encourage clients to pay attention to their skin folds (e.g., groin, axilla) as they can easily become sore if they are not thoroughly dried. This is particularly important for clients who are overweight.

Pay particular attention to clients' feet if they are diabetic or have poor circulation. It is important to clean and dry thoroughly between the toes to prevent fungal infections.

Use toiletries appropriately. For example, ensure that deodorants are not making the skin sore, and avoid using too much talcum powder that can collect in skin crevices and cause soreness.

If you notice any problems with a client's skin (e.g., soreness, discolouration, infections, wounds, ulcers), this should be reported immediately to the person-in-charge.

Care of the Mouth

Three main functions of the mouth are ingestion of food and water, communication, and breathing (in conjunction with the nasal cavity). The lips form the entrance to the mouth cavity which contains the cheeks, gums, tongue, and teeth. The mouth is lubricated by the secretions of the salivary glands (saliva), which protects the mouth and helps to digest food.

The aims of mouth care and oral hygiene include the following:

- Keep the lips and mucosal layer on the inside of the mouth clean, soft, moist, and intact, in order to prevent infection.
- Remove food debris, including dental plaque, without damaging the gums.
- Alleviate pain and discomfort whilst promoting the oral intake of food and fluids.
- Freshen the mouth, and prevent halitosis (bad breath).

Poor oral health can result in mouth ulcers, infection, bleeding gums, dental caries (tooth decay), difficulties in tasting, swallowing, speaking, and respiration. The main factors which tend to cause poor oral health include the following:

- Not taking adequate fluids
- Poor nutritional status
- Insufficient saliva production
- Lack of knowledge or motivation to maintain oral hygiene

Exercise 6.8 🖊

Mouth care includes an oral assessment which should indicate the type of oral care tools and agents that are required. The tools may include toothbrush, foamstick, dental floss, and gauze. Choose the tool that will clean the teeth well without damaging the gums. The toothbrush, in most cases, is the tool of choice. There is a wide choice of oral care agents, depending on whether the main aim is to remove food debris and plaque, prevent infection, alleviate pain, stop bleeding, or provide lubrication. For most people, the agent of choice is toothpaste.

To maintain good oral hygiene, a person needs to clean the teeth with a toothbrush and toothpaste after meals and floss regularly. Sometimes clients are unable to do this for themselves, and you will have to do it for them.

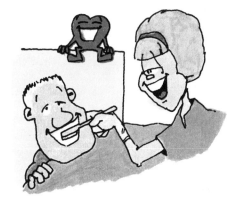

When **brushing teeth**, follow this procedure:

1. Assemble your equipment—plastic cups, waste bowl or sink, towel or paper tissues, soft toothbrush, toothpaste, dental floss, mouthwash.

2. Wash your hands with bacteriocidal soap and water or bacteriocidal alcohol hand rub, and dry with a paper towel.

3. Inform the client what you are going to do, and ensure privacy.

4. If the teeth are to be flossed, do this before brushing. Take care to slide the floss gently between the teeth without damaging the gums, and remember to use a fresh section of floss for each gap between the teeth.

113

5. Hold the toothbrush at a 45 degree angle, and brush the teeth and massage the gums thoroughly, ensuring that you do not press too hard and damage the gums. When brushing the teeth, always brush away from the gums.

6. Brush the person's tongue, if requested.

7. Allow the person to gargle with the mouthwash, if required.

8. Give a beaker of water or mouthwash to the client to rinse his or her mouth and then spit the contents into the waste bowl or sink. Dry the person's mouth.

9. Ensure the person is comfortable before leaving.

10. Remove all used equipment and discard waste.

11. Wash your hands with soap and water or alcohol hand rub, and dry with a paper towel.

12. Report any problems to the person-in-charge.

Exercise 6.9 🖉

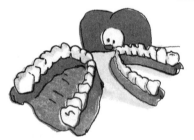

Some people wear full dentures (false teeth), and some wear partial dentures. As a person ages, mouth tissues change, and dentures may need to be replaced. If a client complains of discomfort or develops a sore mouth, notify the person-in-charge.

Remove dentures from the mouth for at least eight hours per day, and store them in water to prevent warping. Assist clients, as needed, to rinse dentures after meals and snacks and to clean them thoroughly once a day. Major problems with dentures include getting them lost or mixed up with other people's dentures.

Therefore, only clean one set of dentures at a time. Take care with the choice of mouth wash as some can affect dentures. For example, ferric chloride, a salivary stimulant, can cause dentures to turn black.

For **denture care**, follow this procedure:

1. Assemble the equipment—basin, denture brush, drinking glass or plastic cup, towel and/or paper tissues, toothbrush.

2. Wash your hands with bacteriocidal soap and water or bacteriocidal alcohol hand rub, and dry with a paper towel.

3. Inform the client what you are going to do, and ensure privacy.

4. Remove the client's dentures using a tissue, and place them in a solution of denture cleaner.

5. With the dentures removed, use the toothbrush to clean the person's remaining teeth (if there are any).

6. Fill the basin with warm (not hot) water, and hold the dentures over the water to avoid breaking them, if they are dropped.

7. Use the denture brush to clean the dentures. They can be left to soak for longer if there are stubborn stains. Never use a sharp tool for cleaning dentures.

8. Store the dentures in water, or insert them into the person's mouth.

9. Ensure the person is comfortable before you leave him or her.

10. Remove all used equipment, and discard waste.

11. Wash your hands with soap and water or alcohol hand rub, and dry with a paper towel.

12. Report any problems to the person-in-charge.

Exercise 6.10 🖉

Extensive mouth care may be necessary for some clients. Occasionally, because of poor oral hygiene or because of illness, a client's mouth can become very dry and dirty, resulting in smelly breath (halitosis) and a mouth infection. More extensive mouth care may also be needed for clients who are unconscious, dehydrated, nauseous and vomiting, nil by mouth, or mouth breathers. Always provide extensive care when a nasogastric tube is in place or if a client is receiving oxygen by an oxygen mask.

Use the following procedure:

1. Assemble your equipment—clinically clean tray, plastic cups, mouthwash or mouth cleaning solution (e.g., chlorhexidine gluconate 0.2 percent diluted in 100 mls of water), waste bowl or sink, paper tissues, wooden spatula, soft toothbrush, toothpaste, gloves, small torch, and denture pot.

2. Wash your hands with bacteriocidal soap and water or bacteriocidal alcohol hand rub, and dry with a paper towel.

3. Prepare the required solution for mouthwash.

4. Inform the client what you are going to do.

5. Where appropriate, remove the client's dentures using a tissue.

6. Inspect the mouth with the aid of a spatula and small torch.

7. Using the toothpaste, gently but firmly brush the teeth, gums, and tongue. When brushing the teeth, always brush away from the gums.

8. Give a beaker of water or mouthwash to the client to rinse the mouth and then spit the contents into the waste bowl or sink.

9. If the client is unable to do this for him/herself, use a rinsed toothbrush on the teeth and moistened foam sticks for the gums and inside of the mouth, using a rotating action so that all the surface area is covered.

10. If necessary, apply artificial saliva to the tongue and a suitable lubricant to dry lips.

11. Clean the dentures on all surfaces using a denture brush or toothbrush and toothpaste.

12. Rinse the dentures, and return them to the client's mouth. If there is an oral infection, the dentures can be soaked in chlorhexidine solution for 10 minutes.

13. Remove all used equipment, and discard waste.

14. Wash your hands with soap and water or alcohol hand rub, and dry with a paper towel.

Exercise 6.11

Care of the Skin

It is important to maintain healthy skin. Skin functions include maintaining temperature, protection, excretion (sweat and sebum), and sensation.

Skin has three layers—epidermis, dermis, and a deep subcutaneous layer. The epidermis is on the outside. The cells on the surface are continually being rubbed off and replaced by new cells which grow from underneath. The epidermis has hairs, sweat glands, and the ducts of sebaceous glands protruding through it.

Exercise 6.12

The initial stage of skin care is to observe the general condition of the skin. Several factors may influence the state of the skin. The level of **hydration** is important. Dehydration will cause the skin to appear inelastic and dry, and oedema (abnormal swelling of tissues due to fluid retention) causes stretching and thinning of the skin. **Age** can affect the level of elasticity in the skin, producing wrinkles and making it more prone to damage. **Health** status (e.g., venous ulcers, pressure sores, wounds), and skin conditions can also affect the health of the skin (e.g., psoriasis, eczema). See Module 5, Part 4, for guidelines on preventing pressure sores.

Any skin problems should prompt you to take extra care during bathing procedures. Remember people's preferences for personal hygiene (e.g., some people do not like soap on their faces, especially if it tends to dry their skin).

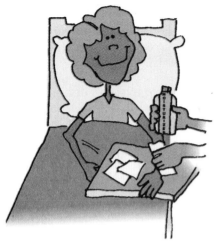

Make sure that people who prefer moisturisers and other creams applied to their skin, have their wishes respected.

Undertake a full assessment before deciding on the type of skin cleansing to use for an individual, and always encourage people to be self-caring, where possible. Provide support and/or equipment, depending on the level of assistance required. In some cultures, people prefer to be cleansed under running water, rather than being sat in a bath.

Always take extra care with skin folds, creases, and crevices. Ensure that they are thoroughly cleaned and dried, and inspected for damage. You will also need to take care when washing and bathing clients who have dressings or intravenous lines. Avoid disturbing dressings/drainage tubes, and keep them dry in order to prevent infection from being introduced to the sites.

Perineal care is the one area of hygiene that is most likely to cause embarrassment and humiliation. It is important to ensure that this area of the body is kept meticulously clean and dry. This is especially important when a client has a problem with this area of the body (e.g., catheter, wound, diarrhoea). Therefore, extreme care should be taken to ensure privacy and minimise embarrassment, taking into account the individual's personal preferences for the care of this area of the body.

Preferably, the personal hygiene of the perineum should take place after having a bath. If having a bed bath, the water should be changed, and different wipes should be used after the perineum has been cleaned. This is important because many micro-organisms live around this area of the body.

Exercise 6.13 🖎

Hair Care

The appearance of a person's hair can have a significant effect on that person's self-esteem. Some people wash and groom their hair every day. Others prefer to leave it alone for days or weeks at a time. Always take the time to find out a client's preferences for hair care.

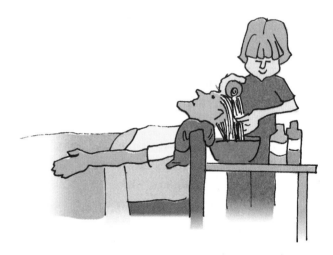

Washing hair is quite an easy task unless a client is confined to bed. Even then, if you can get the client's head to the foot of the bed and hang it over the edge, it is possible to wash the hair. If hair washing is not feasible (e.g., due to a head wound), you can use an aerosol dry shampoo. The ideal situation is to wash hair while the client is in the bath or shower.

Grooming the hair provides a good opportunity to assess the head and scalp for dandruff, wounds, head lice, etc. Some religions insist that hair is neither washed nor brushed, and other religions insist on the hair being covered (e.g., by a turban).

For **hair washing**, follow this procedure:

1. Assemble the equipment—shampoo, conditioner, towel, brush, comb.

2. Wash your hands.

3. Explain what you are going to do, and then take the person to the sink if he or she is not in the bath or shower.

4. If required, brush or comb the hair gently to remove tangles before washing.

5. If required, adjust the position of the person's head in readiness for the hair washing.

6. Adjust the water temperature for the person's comfort.

7. Wet the hair, and apply a small amount of shampoo to the hair.

8. Shampoo the hair gently, massaging the scalp, whilst avoiding getting the shampoo in the person's eyes and ears.

9. Observe for scalp irritation or other problems.

10. Use conditioner, if required by the person.

11. Rinse the person's hair, being careful not to spill water onto the floor or the person's clothes.

12. Rinse and pat the hair dry with a towel. Finish the drying process with a hair dryer.

13. Style the person's hair using a comb and/or brush.

14. Leave the person in a comfortable position.

15. Wash your hands.

16. Report any problems or difficulties to the person-in-charge.

Exercise 6.14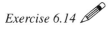

Most people are particular about the way they keep their hair. The accepted hairstyles for men and women range from waist length hair to punk rocker, multi-coloured hair to permed hair, crew cuts to shaven heads. Clients should be allowed to choose their own hairstyles, even if those hairstyles appear to be inappropriate or scruffy to you. Clients should be encouraged to care for their own hair, if they are able. For some clients, their style of hair is the most important aspect of their appearance.

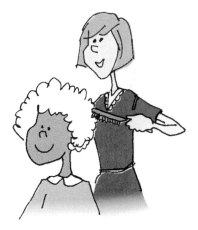

Daily hair care includes brushing and/or combing as often as is necessary to keep the hair in place and to maintain the individual's desired appearance. Use a brush or comb of an appropriate type for the hair care required, and ensure that it is in good condition and clean.

Long hair that is tangled should be combed/brushed one section at a time to prevent damaging the hair and hurting the client. If you are caring for a client from a different ethnic group who has a type of hair or hairstyle that you are not used to caring for, you may need to seek advice on the best way of looking after that client's hair.

If you care for clients from different ethnic minorities, it will be worth your while to find out more information. Read books or ask the clients themselves about their different cultures.

Exercise 6.15 🖉

Remember the hair on other parts of the body. Some women prefer their axilla and other parts of their bodies to remain clean shaven/stubble free. Men may need help with the grooming/shaving of their facial hair.

Shaving is an individual choice. Many males prefer a clean shaven face. Many women prefer to have their legs and underarms shaved. In addition, some women like to have their bikini lines waxed/shaved and their eyebrows plucked. Where appropriate, help the client to undertake these personal grooming tasks.

To shave with an **electric shaver**, follow these guidelines:

1. Wash your hands.

2. Gather the equipment—the client's own electric razor and aftershave or skin lotion (if required).

3. Ask the client's permission, and/or explain what you are going to do.

4. If the client has just had a bath or shower, it may be appropriate to wait until the skin and hair are fully dry as this makes shaving with an electric razor easier.

5. Ensure that the razor is in good working order before you use it. Some care establishments require that all electrical equipment is checked by an electrician for safety, before it can be used.

6. Do not use the razor near a sink or bath as the razor would be ruined if dropped in water. There is also the danger of electrocution if the razor is plugged in. Also, ensure that the razor is not dropped onto the floor as it can break quite easily and is expensive to replace.

7. Follow the manufacturer's instructions when using the razor. Some razors should be moved in small rotating movements on the skin. Others require you to move the razor in a straight line. Make sure that you do not press too hard with the razor, or you may make the skin sore.

8. Some razors have attachments for trimming moustaches and beards. If you use the attachments, make sure you do not trim off too much hair, or you may upset the client.

9. If the razor is not working properly, check that it is plugged in/charged up, is not clogged with hair and needs cleaning out, and does not have components missing or damaged.

10. After shaving, check that the client is satisfied with the end result.

11. Apply aftershave or skin lotion, if required.

12. Clear away the equipment, and clean out the shaver.

13. Wash your hands.

Exercise 6.16 🖉

For a **wet shave**, follow these guidelines:

1. Wash your hands.

2. Gather the equipment—the client's own wet razor, razor blades (if required), towel, wash cloth, shaving cream, aftershave or skin lotion (if required).

3. Ask the client's permission and/or explain what you are going to do.

4. It is usually best to wet shave after bathing when the skin is soft. If necessary, use a warm wash cloth to soften the skin.

5. Apply the shaving cream to the areas of skin to be shaved.

6. When shaving, shave in the direction that the hair grows. You may need to hold the skin taut if it is wrinkled. If you nick the skin, utilise Universal Precautions (see Module 4, Part 2), and apply a small plaster to the cut after the skin has been rinsed and thoroughly dried.

7. After shaving, rinse off any residual shaving cream, dry the area, and apply aftershave or skin lotion, as required.

8. Ensure that the client is comfortable, and check that the client is satisfied with the end result.

9. Clear away the equipment, and rinse out the razor.

10. Wash your hands.

Exercise 6.17 🖉

Personal Grooming and Appearance

Most people have an interest in how they look and how they are viewed by others. Everybody has different tastes in terms of preference for clothing, hairstyles, toiletries, jewelry, etc. These are influenced by a number of factors including current fashions, present mood, level of self-esteem, finances, etc.

Always allow clients to be as independent as possible. Encourage them to express their preferences and make choices in maintaining their appearance and undertaking personal grooming. This will allow them to feel comfortable with their personal images and promotes self-esteem. Facilities for grooming and dressing should be arranged for privacy and comfort.

The support required by the client should be discussed and agreed with him or her, and should be provided in a way that is consistent with the client's personal beliefs, preferences, and plan of care. Encourage clients to keep their own clothing and grooming equipment secure, clean, and in good condition. Where appropriate, significant changes in the client's habits of grooming and dressing should be reported promptly, especially when this might indicate a change in the client's level of ability, and physical or mental health.

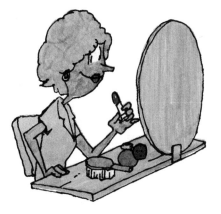

Cosmetics have an important role to play in many people's personal appearance. Personal taste, fashion, and availability are all important factors in the use of cosmetics. Always encourage clients to apply their own cosmetics, whenever possible, and try not to be judgmental. Where appropriate, give honest feedback to your clients on how they look.

A client may choose an appearance that causes problems (e.g., tattoos and body piercing making it more difficult for the client to find a job, tight fitting clothing that is difficult to remove at the toilet, clothing that may give the wrong sexual messages to others, relatives who are likely to be very shocked at the client's appearance). You may have to tentatively broach the subject with the client and offer advice (which may or may not be welcomed and/or accepted) on how to adapt the appearance so that it is less likely to cause problems.

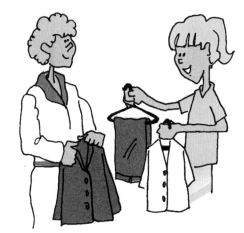

Clothing

Ways in which you can help a client with clothing include helping with purchases, choosing clothing to wear, and dressing and undressing.

Exercise 6.18 🖉

The **selection of clothing** to be worn should take into account a number of factors:

- Personal preferences
- Weather
- Activities that are to be undertaken
- Client's ability to dress/undress
- Whether the clothing is likely to cause problems (e.g., a fastening rubbing the skin and making it sore, difficulties with removing the clothing at the toilet)
- Requirement to wear prostheses/orthoses

Due to illness, disability, or for cosmetic purposes, some clients wear **sensory aids** (e.g., hearing aids, spectacles, voice synthesisers), **prostheses** (e.g., artificial limbs, false eyes, dentures, wigs, false breasts), **orthoses** (e.g., surgical shoes/stockings, callipers, wrist brace, splint, neck brace, corset), or **camouflage creams**.

Be aware that, although sensory aids, prostheses, orthoses, and camouflage creams can be essential for enabling some clients to communicate and undertake the tasks of everyday living, clients can be very sensitive about the need to wear them. The great majority of clients will want to look as "normal" as possible. That is, they want their sensory aids, prosthesis, orthosis, or skin blemishes to remain hidden or be as unobtrusive as possible.

Some clients may need to be encouraged to wear their sensory aids, prosthesis, or orthosis, as indicated in the plan of care. Any concerns relating to their use should be discussed with clients so that an acceptable solution can be found. If you encounter difficulties in supporting a client to wear a sensory aid, prosthesis, orthosis, or camouflage cream, refer the problem to the person-in-charge.

Exercise 6.19

Dressing and undressing can be a problem for some clients due to illness, frailty, or disability. For a client who needs help, explain what you are going to do. Then help the client select appropriate clothing for the activities that are to be undertaken once the client is dressed. Ensure privacy, and always refer to the plan of care.

Do not rush the person into choosing clothes or into getting dressed/undressed. Prepare clothing for dressing or undressing by unbuttoning, unhooking, and unzipping, and ensure that any necessary equipment (e.g., button/zip hook, stocking aid, dressing stick, long shoe horn) is nearby for use by the client.

Clothing should be removed or put on, one piece at a time. You may need to ask which order the client prefers the clothes to be put on. If the client has any physical disabilities or behavioural problems, this may dictate the way that the clothing has to be put on or taken off. For example, if a person cannot use one arm, that arm is placed into clothing first and removed from clothing last. Another example is where a client is likely to kick out at you; do not kneel down to put the client's shoes on if that makes you an easy target for a kick.

Ensure that clothing is worn in an appropriate manner. You will have to decide whether to inform the client if the choice of clothing is not appropriate. Check that clothing has been put on properly and is not rolled up under the client or likely to make the client feel uncomfortable. With the client's permission, fasten any buttons, zips, or other fastenings that have been forgotten. Where appropriate, help the client to "smarten up" (e.g., tuck the shirt in, straighten the tie).

Where appropriate, ask the client to look in the mirror to check his or her appearance. If the client is unable to see for him/herself, provide feedback on how the person looks. All discarded clothing should be folded up and put back into the drawers/wardrobe or placed in the dirty washing basket. Before leaving, make sure that the client is comfortable and happy with the end result.

Exercise 6.20

Nail Care

Although nails can be difficult to keep clean, encourage clients to care for their own nails as much as possible. Always check with the plan of care before giving nail care. If the service is available, a manicure can greatly add to a client's feelings of well-being.

For the care of **fingernails**, follow these guidelines:

1. Wash your hands, and, if necessary, ask the client to wash his or her hands. If appropriate, ask the client to use a nail brush to scrub his or her fingernails.

2. Assemble the equipment—nail scissors/clippers, nail file, emery board, towel, nail polish (if required).

3. Ask the client's permission to provide nail care, and inform the client what you intend to do.

4. If the nails are very thick and tough, you may need to soak them in warm water first to soften them.

5. Place the person's hand on the towel to collect the cut fingernails.

6. Trim the fingernails carefully with the nail scissors/clippers so that they are rounded, making sure that there are no rough edges.

7. Clean the nails of debris with the nail file, and smooth the edges of the nail with an emery board.

8. If required, apply hand lotion and nail polish, and ensure the client is happy with the end result.

9. Clean away the equipment, carefully disposing of the nail clippings and filings.

10. Wash your hands.

Take special care with toenails. Many people have misshapen toes and toenails. Some toenails can be very difficult to cut, requiring the specialist equipment of a chiropodist. For clients who have problems with peripheral circulation (due to diabetes for example), it is usually safer to have their toenails cut by a chiropodist. When their toes are damaged, there is often a significant delay in the healing process.

For **toenails**, the procedure is similar to that for fingernails, with the following exceptions:

- Hand cream will not be applied.

- You will need to use appropriate nail trimmers/cutters that can cope with thick toenails.

- The toenails should be cut straight across, not rounded.

- Report any foot problems (e.g., corns, calluses, ingrowing toenails, ulcers, infections) to the person-in-charge so that a chiropodist or doctor can be called in to treat them.

Exercise 6.21 🖉

Part 2: Eating and Drinking (Z10)

Encourage health and well-being by enabling others to eat and drink.

Care organisations differ in their provisions for ensuring that clients are well nourished. Even when clients are very ill, it is important that they receive some nourishment to encourage healing or prevent deterioration of their condition. Therefore, this is an important aspect of care that ensures the health and well-being of the clients in your care.

Health and Diet

There are six basic rules for healthy eating—natural foods; high in fibre; low in sugar, salt, and fat; and enough calories to maintain weight.

Natural foods (not refined) are important because the refining process removes a lot of the goodness out

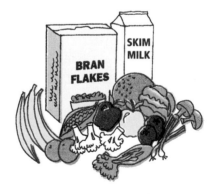

of the food (e.g., white bread, canned vegetables). A number of preservatives, additives, and dyes are often added to the food to ensure that it does not deteriorate and to make it more presentable to the consumer (e.g., cooked meats, some soft drinks).

Foods that are **high in fibre** make you feel full, contain few calories, and help to prevent constipation.

Foods that are **low in sugar** provide healthier eating because sweet foods only stem your hunger for a very short period of time before you have a craving for more. Although sugar is an easy source of energy, it provides few vitamins and minerals and is, therefore, not required within the diet.

Foods that are **low in salt** help to prevent problems in people who are susceptible to developing high blood pressure. The salt that occurs naturally in food is enough to meet daily requirements. It is better to use spices and herbs, rather than salt, to flavour food.

Foods that are **low in fat** help prevent health problems. Fat is high in calories, and animal (saturated) fats from dairy products, lard, and fatty meats have a tendency to result in heart disease in later life. Therefore, when fat is part of a meal, it is better if the fat is vegetable (polyunsaturated) in origin as seen in olive oil and many margarines.

People need enough calories to keep their weight relatively constant and to avoid being significantly overweight or underweight. People who are very overweight or underweight have a greater tendency to become ill, especially if they are not very fit.

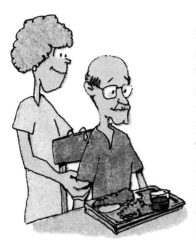

Keep these rules in mind at meal times, and achieve a balanced diet that provides all the necessary foodstuffs, vitamins, minerals, and fluids that are needed. These are essential for keeping teeth, bones, skin, heart, and the other parts of the body in good condition.

Exercise 6.22

Keep to a relatively healthy diet, and maintain your weight within acceptable limits for yourself so that you may advise a client on dietary intake without appearing hypocritical.

All care organisations have to ensure that their clients have access to nutritious diets. This can be difficult as the catering department will be expected to provide hot and cold food of a high quality, at specific times of the day, to meet a wide range of tastes and dietary needs. A range of foods should be available to meet clients' normal dietary needs.

It is expected that any care organisation, even the smallest residential facility, can meet individual dietary requirements. This includes a menu pattern that changes on a regular basis so that the food does not become boring to long-term clients. It also means the availability of different foods each meal time so that there is client choice, and the clients have the opportunity to change their minds. The catering department must be willing to cater for the special dietary needs of any client that the care facility has chosen to accept.

Exercise 6.23

Encouraging Healthier Diets

Most people's dietary habits and current eating patterns are formed over many years. This process starts as children when they develop likes and dislikes for food in the family home, and it continues during their lifetimes where it is adapted by fashion, lifestyle, available money, personal experiences, peer group pressure, culture, religion, etc. This process can result in some individuals having very fixed eating habits and strong opinions about diets and dieting, which can result in some problems.

Some clients will not change their diets just because you tell them to. They may feel that you are making a personal attack on them if you describe their diets as unhealthy or accuse them of eating "risky" foods. If you are working with older people, you have to ask yourself if it is fair to ask them to significantly change their diets at this stage of their lives. It can also be very difficult to deny sweets, chocolate, crisps, and other "goodies" to children.

Unless clients have to change their diets so that they do not become ill (e.g., due to diabetes), the best way to encourage them to eat healthier diets is to emphasise the "pay-offs" that they are likely to get. The reasons that you can use to help encourage clients to eat healthier diets might include any of the following:

- A healthy diet can help to achieve a good complexion by helping to clear up spots.

- A healthy diet would result in a reduction in weight so you can fit into all those clothes in your wardrobe that are too small at the moment.

- A healthy diet often makes people feel healthier and have more energy.

- A healthier diet means an introduction to a new world of tasty dishes.

- A healthy diet is an essential component of preparation for any sportsman or athlete.

- Choosing more natural foods for children avoids all the food additives (colourings and preservatives) that make certain children hyperactive.

- Increasing fibre intake helps to prevent constipation and relieves piles.

- Eating less sugary foods can reduce your calorie intake and help to avoid tooth decay.

- For some people, eating less can result in a lowered blood pressure.

Exercise 6.24

Clients will normally have some choice in the food that is prepared for them when at home. When in a care organization, a range of people may be involved in selecting the foods that are available. They may include the following:

- Dietitians
- Care staff
- Speech therapist
- Catering manager
- Rehabilitation therapist
- Doctors

A large care organisation will have a wide range of different diets every day. Following are examples:

- Soft diets containing only soft and liquid or semi-liquid foods that are easy to swallow for people who have mouth problems or difficulties with swallowing

- Vegetarian diets for clients who do not eat meat

- Diets to meet religious and cultural requirements (e.g., the provision of Halal meat for Moslems)

- Reducing diets for clients who need to reduce weight (e.g., 1,000-1,500 calorie diets)

- Diets that avoid certain foods (e.g., nuts) because the client has an allergy to them

Some client groups have specific dietary requirements. Following are examples:

Muslims are not allowed to eat pork or pork products, and all other meat that is eaten must be Halal (killed in a specific way). Alcohol is strictly prohibited. During the month of Ramadan, Muslims are expected to fast.

Hindus are often vegetarians as they feel it is wrong to kill animals for food. The cow is considered to be a sacred beast and, therefore, eating beef is strictly prohibited. Many Hindus also refuse alcohol.

Sikhs will usually refuse beef and alcohol.

Jews do not eat any pig meats (e.g., pork, ham, bacon), and they have rules about the way animals should be killed for meat and in the preparation of food.

Catholics may prefer to eat only fish on Fridays.

Methodists are prohibited alcohol.

Vegetarians do not eat any meat or fish.

Vegans are strict vegetarians. They also do not eat any dairy or animal produce (e.g., eggs, milk, cheese, yoghurt).

Exercise 6.25

Individual clients should not be stereotyped because of their beliefs, religion, or culture. Individuals from these groups may not strictly follow the dietary restrictions, especially if they have lived in this country for many years. Therefore, you should not automatically presume that you know what these clients want to eat and drink. Always ask clients for their preferences. Do not be surprised to find individuals from these groups occasionally prefer a Big Mac to a curry or nut cutlet.

A wide range of special diets may also be available to accommodate specific health issues. Examples include diabetic, high fibre, bland, fat free, and low protein.

Diabetic diets are usually sugar-free. Only measured quantities of carbohydrates are given to clients.

High fibre diets include lots of fresh fruits and vegetables and high fibre foods. These are often provided to clients who have bowel problems (e.g., constipation).

Bland diets are simple foods, sometimes only given in small amounts, that are easily digested (e.g., milk pudding, toast). They are often provided to clients who have digestion problems or who have been vomiting.

Fat-free diets are usually provided as part of a calorie-controlled diet or for clients who have gall bladder and digestion problems.

Low protein diets are usually provided for clients who have kidney problems.

Exercise 6.26

Indigestion is a common problem. It normally occurs because the stomach's gastric acid irritates the lining of the stomach wall or the oesophagus. Always report indigestion to the person-in-charge as the main symptom for a heart attack may be acute indigestion.

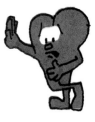

Nausea and vomiting can occur when food or drink that has been swallowed makes the client feel unwell. This may simply be one of the symptoms of an illness from which the client is suffering, or it may be something unexpected like food poisoning.

When a client vomits, the first priority is to make sure that the client does not choke by inhaling the vomit. Therefore, the person should be leaned forward so that all vomit can easily exit the body. Nausea and vomiting should always be reported/recorded immediately.

Food allergies can occur when a client has an allergic reaction to a food or component of food or drink that has been eaten. Usually you will be aware that a client has a food allergy, as that information is requested as part of the initial assessment of a client. Sometimes you may not know about a client's food allergy, or the client may develop a new food allergy.

The allergic reaction can vary from just a simple rash on the client's chest to a severe allergic reaction (often referred to as anaphylactic shock) where the client's body is quickly covered in a rash and the throat swells up, blocking off the airway. This can result in death if not treated very quickly. Therefore, all allergic reactions to food and drink should be immediately reported to the person-in-charge.

Monitoring Intake of Food and Drink

There are many reasons why it is necessary to monitor a client's intake of food and drink:

- To ensure an adequate intake of fluids (e.g., in order to prevent a client from becoming

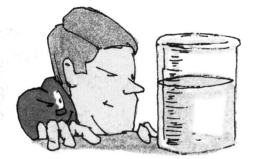

that it loses when there is a shortage, and it can increase the excretion of water from the body when the intake is too high. The correct amount of water is needed by the body to maintain the concentration of electrolytes both inside and outside of the billions of cells that make up the human body.

When a person becomes **dehydrated**, you will see the following signs:

- The skin becomes dry and inelastic. When it is pinched, it does not quickly regain its shape.

- The person feels thirsty.

- The mouth will be very dry, and the tongue may be coated.

- The urine becomes very concentrated, and output drops to a minimum.

- The person may become disorientated; if the dehydration continues, he or she may die.

A person can also retain water in the form of **oedema** (tissue swelling). There are a large number of potential causes of oedema, but the following signs are usually present:

- Some parts of the body will swell because water has been retained.

- There will be weight gain.

- In generalised oedema, the water eventually settles, due to gravity, in the lowest parts of the body (e.g., the ankles for a person who is stood up, the back and buttocks for someone who is laid in bed).

When monitoring fluid balance, ensure that you measure (or estimate, if necessary) and record all fluids going into a client (e.g., drinks, intravenous fluids), and all fluids that come out of a client (e.g., urine, faeces, vomit, drainage from a wound).

Exercise 6.28

dehydrated or to ensure that toxins are flushed out of the body)

- When fluid balance (intake and output of fluids) has to be strictly monitored (e.g., when a client has oedema, for kidney disease)

- When a client's calorie intake has to be carefully monitored (when he or she is overweight or underweight)

- When a client is on a special diet as part of the plan of care, and you need to ensure that the diet is being adhered to

- To ensure that a balanced diet is being consumed as part of the plan of care when the client has certain psychological problems (e.g., bulimia where the client may eat the meal and then go to the toilet to vomit in order to stay slim)

Exercise 6.27

In many care environments, one of the most important aspects of monitoring what a client consumes is the recording of fluids using a **fluid balance** chart. The human body is more than 90 percent water. It constantly loses water and, therefore, must have a constant supply of water to replenish the reservoir. Water is lost from the body in urine, faeces, sweat, vomit, and during respiration.

Water can be gained by the body naturally in food and drink or artificially by intravenous infusion. The body can reduce (but not stop) the amount of water

The following approximate measures in millilitres (mls) are only a guide to the quantity of fluid that has been consumed by a client:

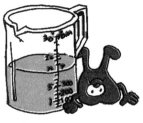

- A sip = 10 mls
- A glass = 190 mls
- A cup = 150 mls
- A mug = 290 mls
- Plastic jug = 850 mls
- 120 grams of custard = 90 mls

To get an accurate measure of **fluid intake**, it is necessary to record all the fluids the client drinks or that are intravenously infused into the client. Explain to the client what you are doing and why you are doing it. You will need the client's cooperation to ensure that no fluids are consumed that are not entered onto the fluid balance chart. You will also need to measure foods such as ice cream, jelly, and custard. Be sure to record intake as soon as it is consumed.

To get an accurate measure of **fluid output**, it is necessary to record all the fluids that come out of a client. Drainage bottles and the contents of catheter bags are easily measured. Other fluid outputs (e.g., in faeces and when someone has vomited over the floor) have to be estimated. One simple ploy is to remind the client to tell you when he or she wants to use the toilet.

Report all problems relating to fluid balance measurement to the person-in-charge.

Exercise 6.29 🖊

Helping Clients to Eat and Drink

Most people have a great deal of control over when, where, and what they eat. Illness, disability, or learning difficulty may result in some clients having less control over their eating and drinking arrangements.

Exercise 6.30 🖊

All equipment used for eating, drinking, and the feeding of others should be scrupulously clean to prevent cross-infection. Some foods need to be maintained at a certain temperature so that they remain edible, do not deteriorate, and cannot cause harm or discomfort to clients.

Where possible, always involve clients in the process of choosing their own food and drink, and if possible, negotiate with clients the level of support (if any) required to eat and drink. Some clients may want drinks or snacks at times other than meal times.

Also, where possible, allow clients to choose where and how they eat (e.g., standing at a burger bar, holding fish and chips in paper on the lap, lying on the floor in front of the television, or sitting on the grass having a picnic). Always provide clients with a choice of feeding utensils. Where appropriate, care staff and clients should eat together to reduce the feeling of "them and us," and so that feeding and personal skills can be taught to others in an informal way.

Where appropriate, include relatives and friends in helping the client to eat and drink. This can have a great psychological benefit for both the client and significant others. Try to make meal times leisurely and relaxed, and avoid being judgmental of clients in terms of what they eat and the way that they eat (e.g., table manners). Questions relating to diet posed by clients and/or their families which are beyond your care role, should be promptly referred to a more experienced member of the care team.

Exercise 6.31 🖊

Some clients will require help in **preparing for meal times** so that they feel comfortable and relaxed before and during the meal. Always allow clients the choice of going to the toilet and the opportunity to wash their hands and face before the meal. Some clients may require oral hygiene care before eating. Some may require their dentures to be cleaned and put comfortably in place in preparation for the meal.

If required, help clients to get to the eating area. Some clients prefer a set place at a table and may become upset if they are forced to sit in another place.

Where appropriate, clients should be positioned so that they can interact at meal times in order that meal times can become a social occasion. Those clients who need help with feeding should be placed so that care staff can easily access them.

If required, enable the client to be comfortably positioned in an upright manner to help with the swallowing of food. For those clients who cannot sit upright because of illness or disability, check their plans of care for the most comfortable eating position.

Ensure that clients have protection for their clothing (e.g., paper napkins), or items of clothing may need to be removed before eating and replaced afterwards.

Exercise 6.32

Some clients have difficulty in feeding themselves. This can happen for a number of reasons. For example, the client is unable to use the upper limbs due to paralysis or serious illness, the client's upper limb coordination has been lost due to physical or mental illness, the client has recently lost his or her eyesight, the client has injuries to the mouth area, the client is very frail, the client has not yet learned to feed him/herself properly. Therefore, some clients will require practical assistance with eating and drinking.

The amount of help that is given to a client at meal times depends on what the client can do for him/herself. Some clients are able to do almost everything for themselves as long as they have the right equipment. Other clients may need a lot more help—positioning, cutting food, feeding, ensuring that choking does not occur, wiping mouths and chins, etc. In fact, some clients will require you to do everything for them apart from chewing and swallowing the food.

Exercise 6.33

Some clients require **aids for eating and drinking**. Examples include specially shaped or adapted cutlery with and without finger yokes, adapted meal trays designed to hold plates and utensils securely, suction or non-slip pads for plates and dishes, suction egg cups to enable a person with one hand to eat a boiled egg, dishes that have boiling water in the base to keep the food hot, specially partitioned plates, plate surrounds which snap onto plates, special drinking vessels (with lids, spouts, or straws) with a variety of different handles.

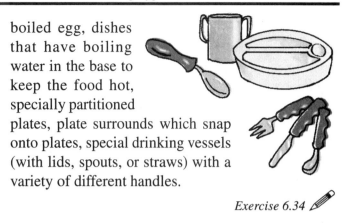

Exercise 6.34

To feed a dependent client, prepare the client for eating and drinking—position him or her, provide opportunities for toileting, wash hands and face, etc. Collect together all the necessary equipment onto the trolley or tray, including feeding utensils such as cutlery, drinking cup with spout or angled straw; paper napkin or towel; and receptacle for soiled, disposable equipment.

Explain what you are going to do so that you can get the client's informed consent and cooperation. If necessary, provide an explanation for the equipment and feeding technique that you intend to use. Serve the client's food as ordered, according to the plan of care.

If there is not enough room to feed the client, with the client's permission, make room for yourself and your equipment. Sit where you can observe the client and interact with him or her during the meal. Where appropriate, sit with or near other clients who are eating.

You may need to remind the client of what was ordered on the menu, especially if the client is blind and cannot see the food. If the ordered food and drink are not acceptable, try to offer alternatives. Ask the client which food he or she would prefer to eat first.

Always keep food covered until it is ready to be served or eaten. This keeps it warm, stops it from drying out, and prevents insects from landing on it. Make condiments (e.g., salt and pepper) and garnishes (e.g., mustard, horseradish, sauces, relishes) available.

When the client has finished eating and drinking, if necessary, restore the client's physical environment back to its original condition. Clear away the used equipment, dispose of any waste, and wash your hands.

If required, make a record of the food and drink that has been consumed and any other relevant facts that need to be reported. You may be required to monitor the after effects of the meal on the client (e.g., client is still hungry/thirsty, feels overfull, nausea or vomiting).

Follow these specific guidelines for feeding a dependent client:

1. Wash your hands thoroughly (preferably with bacteriocidal soap and water or bacteriocidal hand rub).

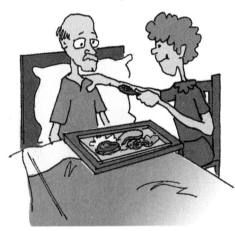

2. Provide any necessary support to enable the client to maintain an upright position at meal times. The client may have to be repositioned if he or she slides out of position during the feeding process.

3. Ensure that the food is not too hot or too cold and that the food remains at a suitable temperature. Some clients will want to check the temperature of the food before the feeding process commences.

4. The food should be offered to the client at a pace that is dictated by the client. Avoid feeding the client too quickly as this could result in choking.

5. Carefully place the fork or spoon in the client's mouth to prevent injuries to the mouth, teeth, and gums and to prevent gagging or choking when the fork or spoon has been pushed too far into the client's mouth.

6. Where appropriate, assist the client to feed him/herself, even when spillages are likely, so that he or she can eventually become less dependent on others.

7. Clean up any spillages at the earliest opportunity, and replace spilled food and drink.

8. A client who has lost the feeling or movement on one side of the face may need to be fed to one side of the mouth only. Take care to ensure that food does not accumulate in the other side of the mouth.

9. If required, the client should be provided with sips of fluid during the meal to aid swallowing and for the cleansing of the palate prior to a change of food.

10. Closely observe the client during the feeding process for signs of discomfort, distaste, choking, or simply that the client has had enough. If the client appears to be choking, sit him or her slightly forward to facilitate clearing the mouth of food.

11. Before leaving the client, make sure that he or she is clean, tidy, and comfortable. Some clients may require mouth care after they have been fed (especially if food tends to collect in the mouth) to maintain oral hygiene. Also, some clients will want the opportunity to wash their hands and face and/or brush their teeth.

Exercise 6.35 🖉

Part 3: Using Toilet Facilities (Z11)

Provide access, comfort, and privacy for use of toilet facilities.

Elimination or excretion is the body's natural way of getting rid of waste products and is essential for the body to function properly. In the normal expectation of a lifetime, it is acceptable for all babies to be incontinent. Their bladders and bowels fill and empty automatically. By the age of three years, it is expected that most children will be fully continent during the day and, by the age of five years, most will also be continent during the night. They learn the feeling of bladder and bowel fullness and to link this to the need to use the toilet or hold the contents until a toilet is available. Good bladder and bowel control are normally expected to be maintained throughout life, although it is accepted that in old age there may be degenerative changes in the body which affect personal elimination.

Elimination Problems

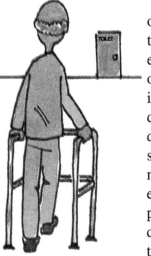

Unfortunately, not everyone finds it easy to access the toilet. The toilets may not be easily accessible or available, or the client may have mobility problems making it difficult to get to the toilet quickly. The client may be positioned a long way from the nearest toilet, or the physical environment may cause a problem (e.g., stairs, narrow doorways, blocked corridors, toilet too high or too low).

When there is a lack of privacy and/or toilet door locks are not secure, this can put people off using the toilet. Access to, and ability to use, toilet paper is an important aspect of toileting if soiled undergarments are to be avoided.

Exercise 6.36 🖉

In a care facility, access to toilets should not be a problem, but the thought of having to use communal toilets makes many people feel uncomfortable. The toilets may not seem clean enough or smell nice enough. The thought of someone using the toilet next to you can cause uneasiness, especially if that person might be someone of the opposite sex and/or can hear and smell everything that is going on.

Exercise 6.37 🖉

The problem is exacerbated when commodes, sani-chairs, bedpans, and urinals need to be used. Some clients cope very well with this form of toileting. For others, the stress of toileting in this fashion is likely to make them upset and affect their normal patterns of elimination. It is up to you to negotiate a mutually acceptable solution to toileting problems with the client and/or the family.

Drugs which are taken for physical illnesses can affect bladder and/or bowel function. One example is diuretics which substantially increase urine output and can result in incontinence if there are mobility problems. Other categories of drugs used to treat illnesses (e.g., pain, respiratory, cardiac and psychological problems), can affect smooth muscle in other parts of the body causing frequency/retention of urine and/or constipation/diarrhoea. An example here is opiates which are used to combat severe pain. They frequently cause constipation and severe faecal impaction by lowering bowel motility.

When talking about elimination, urine and faeces are the waste products that usually come to mind. But, they can be accompanied by blood, mucus, pus, etc. Therefore, when dealing with *all* body waste products (e.g., blood, vomit), remember to use Universal Precautions. (See Module 4, Part 2.)

Bowel Problems

Diarrhoea can be defined as an abnormal increase in the frequency, quantity, and fluid content of faeces which can be accompanied by urgency, perianal and/or abdominal discomfort, and incontinence. The main treatment is to identify and treat the cause of the diarrhoea.

- *Acute diarrhoea* can be caused by, for example, food poisoning, bowel-irritating diets (e.g., excessive spices, fruit, beer), allergies to certain food constituents.
- *Chronic diarrhoea* can be caused by, for example, drugs (e.g., antibiotics), diseases of the colon (e.g., cancer,), inflammatory diseases of the bowel (e.g., Crohn's disease).

The main danger is that a person can become very dehydrated due to diarrhoea, especially if that individual is also vomiting. When somebody is severely constipated, the faecal impaction can cause fluid to leak around the sides of the faeces and cause diarrhoea.

Exercise 6.38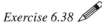

Constipation can be defined as an irregular and infrequent bowel movement associated with the passage of hard, bulky faeces. A client will normally complain of difficulty when defaecating, together with pain and discomfort.

Encopresis refers to incontinence of faeces, usually referring to children who mess their beds at night. By the time a child is five years old, it is usually no longer a problem. If it continues, investigations should be undertaken to try and establish the cause.

Haemorrhoids can make defaecation uncomfortable and/or painful. They sometimes remain in the rectum, but can be forced through the anus with the passage of faeces. When this occurs, they usually have to be manhandled back into the rectum. There are a number of problems that can be caused by haemorrhoids. For example, they can drop through the anus during the day and stain underclothes with faeces or blood, and they can make defaecation painful.

Urinary Problems

The **rate of flow** of urine varies between different people. Some individuals find it very difficult to pass urine anywhere except in their own toilets where they can have quiet and privacy. For others, feelings of apprehensiveness can affect the flow of urine.

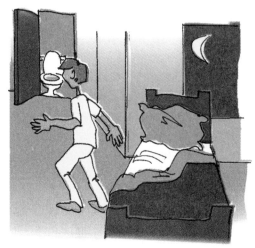

Most people can sleep through the night without having to pass urine. However it is not uncommon, especially for the elderly, to have to pass urine one or more times in the night. This is referred to as **nocturia**. Obviously this affects the amount and quality of sleep a person gets.

Sexual intercourse can also cause problems for the female, especially if there has been a lack of vaginal lubrication. This can lead to cystitis, which makes the bladder very sensitive and leads to frequency and urgency of the need to pass urine.

The most common type of urinary incontinence is the one caused by the feeling that the bladder is overflowing and about to burst. Everyone has experienced the need to "make a run for it." It is characterised by people looking uncomfortable, shuffling their feet, crossing and uncrossing their legs, looking for an opportunity to make a discrete exit, whilst they try to "hold on." If a toilet isn't found in time or their legs "hold on." If a toilet isn't found in time or their legs cannot carry them fast enough, the inevitable leakage of urine occurs. This is called **frequency** or **urge incontinence**. It is often caused by having a small bladder, by the irritation of the bladder wall caused by cystitis, or because an individual has not trained the bladder to hold at least half a pint of urine.

Exercise 6.39

Stress incontinence occurs when the urethral sphincters are not working properly and allow urine to leak, especially during periods of physical exertion which raise intra-abdominal pressure (e.g., lifting, bending, coughing, sneezing, or laughing). It is more common in females, especially those who have some damage to pelvic floor muscles from a prolonged childbirth. For many people who are otherwise fit, healthy, and active, continence can often be restored by retraining and strengthening bladder control.

Outflow obstruction usually involves the neck of the bladder. It is typified by the elderly man with chronic retention of urine who has poor urine flow, even when straining. It is usually caused by enlargement of the prostate gland, tumours in the bladder neck, or sexually transmitted diseases.

Enuresis usually refers to a child wetting the bed. This should no longer be a problem by the time a child is five years old. If it continues, investigations should be undertaken to try and establish the cause. Treatment can include the use of drugs which are given to act on the smooth muscle of the bladder so that there is less likelihood of leakage.

Exercise 6.40

Monitoring Elimination

The assessment of clients' elimination patterns may involve a number of health and social care professionals. When dealing with clients who have elimination problems, the first thing that usually needs to be done is to help them get over their embarrassment when talking about toileting and continence problems. Some clients may become even more embarrassed if a care worker of the same gender is not available with whom they can discuss their problems. Offer them the choice of waiting until a care worker of the same gender is available to talk to them about their elimination needs.

The embarrassment about toileting can be seen in the language that people use. There are many different expressions for emptying the bladder. For example, most people will not use the terms micturition or urination. Instead, they tend to use more colloquial terms (e.g., "passing water," "taking a leak," "doing a number one," or "spending a penny"). There are also many expressions for emptying the bowels (e.g., "taking a dump," "doing a number two," "dropping off a package," or "having a crap").

When talking to clients about their elimination problems, it is important that you talk to them at their level and speed, using words that they understand. Choose your words carefully to ensure that an individual client understands and is not offended or embarrassed.

Exercise 6.41

A full assessment of elimination patterns and/or continence will include asking questions about all the following issues:

- What is the client's general medical history?
- Has the diet and fluid intake been assessed?
- Does the client have a balanced diet with adequate fluids?
- Does the client have easy access to a toilet?
- Does the client have the physical capabilities to dress, undress, and use a toilet?
- Are toileting aids used?
- What are the client's and family's attitudes to the continence problem?
- When did the incontinence commence, and was it connected with any single event?
- Are incontinence aids being used?
- Passing urine:
  - Is the stream good?
  - Are there dribbles after passing urine?

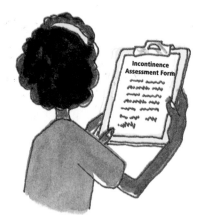

- Passing faeces:
  - Are there haemorrhoids?
- Passing faeces/urine:
  - Does the output look normal?
  - How often?
  - How much?
  - Any leakage?
  - Any pain or discomfort?
  - Is there leakage on coughing, sneezing, or physical exertion?
  - Can the client hold on, or does the toilet have to be accessed quickly?
- At night:
  - Does the client have to use the toilet?
  - How many times?
  - Is there incontinence?
- Physical examinations:
  - Palpation of the abdomen
  - Genitals, perineum, and anus
  - Residual urine
  - Rectal examination
- Has the urine and/or faeces been tested?
- How does the incontinence affect the client's lifestyle?

Exercise 6.42 🖉

Enabling Others to Use the Toilet

For most people, using the toilet is a very private function. Individuals who need help with toileting are likely to find this very embarrassing. It is your job to be professional, to provide privacy, to minimise anxiety, and to maintain the person's dignity throughout the elimination process.

The toilet is the usual place where most people go to pass urine (micturate) or to open their bowels (defaecate). Encourage clients to be as self-managing as possible. Some clients will need varying amounts of assistance and support. Your assistance should be respectful, sensitive to the individual's personal preferences and beliefs, and consistent with the plan of care.

Follow these general guidelines for **toilet use**:

1. Agree with the client the preferred method by which the client can indicate that he or she needs to use toilet facilities.

2. Always allow the client to choose the toilet facility to be used, based on what is available and on the plan of care.

3. Check with the client (and the plan of care, if necessary) whether or not your assistance is required.

4. Always ensure that the client can call for help, if needed, and that the call for help will be answered promptly.

5. Ensure that the client has the necessary materials and/or assistance for cleansing him/herself after using the toilet facilities.

6. If required, ensure that an air freshener spray is made available for clients to mask any smells.

7. Enable the client to wash his or her hands.

8. Ensure that the toilet facilities are clean and tidy for the next person.

9. Thoroughly wash your hands (preferably with bacteriocidal soap and water or bacteriocidal hand rub).

10. Discuss with the client any problems that he or she is having in using the toilet facilities.

11. Report any abnormalities in the client's waste products to an appropriate person at the earliest opportunity. You may want to delay disposing of the waste products until a more experienced member of care staff has seen them.

Exercise 6.43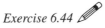

Bedpans, commodes, and urinals can be used for elimination when clients are too ill or too frail to use the toilet, are confined to bed, or are only allowed up for short periods. A separate area should be designated for the storage and disposal of equipment used for toileting, and appropriate hand washing facilities should be made available for both clients and care staff. All toileting equipment should be washed and dried immediately after use.

Ensure that clients know how to call a member of staff when they need to use a toilet facility. Good communication skills by the care worker can prevent clients from having to worry about toilet arrangements (e.g., availability and use of call buttons). Respond immediately when a client needs to use, or has finished using, a toilet facility. Always respond in an appropriate manner—do not show boredom or distaste for the task in hand.

Make sure that the client is as comfortable as possible when using, and after using, toilet facilities. Always ensure as much privacy as possible for the client, especially when this need has to be balanced against the need for safety (e.g., a danger that the client may fall). Where appropriate, offer toilet facilities and hand washing to clients who are not self-caring, prior to meal times.

Exercise 6.44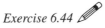

The **bedpan** is a container on which clients can sit and use as a toilet. All bedpans are taken to the bedside and removed from the bedside under a disposable cover. The bedpan can be disposable or non-disposable.

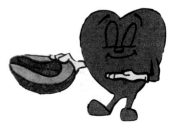

Disposable bedpans are usually placed in a rigid, plastic bedpan holder before being placed under a client. They are disposed of in a bedpan disposal machine that mashes up and swills away the disposable bedpan and its contents. After use, the bedpan holder is usually washed and dried before it is stored. They are sterilised on a regular basis, according to local policies.

Non-disposable bedpans are usually made of stainless steel. They are warmed under hot water and dried before they are used by a client. Used bedpans are placed in a bedpan washer, where they are flushed and washed according to the manufacturer's instructions. Each bedpan is then dried and stored, ready for the next use. Bedpans are sterilised on a regular basis, according to local policies.

Bedpans are used for clients who are confined to their beds. For female clients, bedpans are used for micturition and defaecation. For males, they are used for defaecation only, and a urinal is used for micturition.

Use this procedure when **giving a client a bedpan**:

1. Wash your hands.

2. Collect together all the necessary equipment—bedpan, disposable cover, toilet paper, plastic apron, and gloves.

3. Put on the plastic apron and gloves, and take the covered bedpan to the client's bed.

4. Explain what you are going to do so that you can get the client's consent and cooperation. If necessary, also explain why you intend to do it that way.

5. Help the client into a comfortable position for using the bedpan.

   • Help the client to adjust clothing, continence aids, and appliances so that the buttocks are exposed.

   • Encourage the client to lift the buttocks so that the bedpan can be put in place. Alternatively, log roll the client onto the bedpan, or use a hoist.

   • If required, adjust the client's pillows and raise the bed sides.

   • Ensure that the client is covered for warmth and privacy whilst using the bedpan.

6. Leave the client to use the bedpan, with the toilet tissue nearby if the client can cleanse him/herself after using the bedpan. Ensure that the call button, if available, is within easy reach.

7. Ensure privacy throughout the activity, and make sure you are in the vicinity so that you are available when the client has finished.

8. Do not try to hurry the client who is using the bedpan, although you should not leave anyone on the bedpan for more than 10 minutes.

9. Assist with wiping the client's anal and genital areas, if required. For female clients, ensure that you always wipe from front to back, away from the urethra, with the paper being renewed each wipe. This prevents bacteria from the anus being transferred to the urethra and causing a urinary infection.

10. Remove the bedpan, and place a cover over it.

11. Clean any spillages immediately and thoroughly to prevent accidents and cross-infection.

12. Before leaving, make sure that the client is comfortable.

13. Before disposing of the bedpan, observe the contents and report any abnormalities. If required, measure and test the specimen of urine.

14. When you have disposed of the used bedpan, give the client the opportunity to wash his or her hands.

15. Dispose of the gloves, and wash your hands thoroughly (preferably with bacteriocidal soap and water or bacteriocidal hand rub).

16. Report any problems that the client experienced when using the bedpan.

Note that steps 11-16 listed for bedpans also apply after using commodes and urinals.

Exercise 6.45 ✎

The **commode** is a chair on wheels that has been designed to hold a bedpan in the correct position under the client so that it can be used at the bedside. Some commodes are designed to enable the client to be wheeled to the toilet so that the 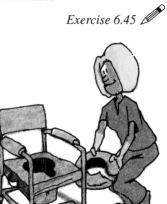 commode can be pushed over the toilet (occasionally referred to as a sanichair). Often a commode is used when a client finds it too uncomfortable or too stressful to use a bedpan.

The procedure for enabling a client to use a commode is essentially the same as that for the bedpan, except that the client has to be helped out of bed and onto the commode first, using safe manual handling techniques. Remember to put the wheel brakes on before the client gets onto the commode. Check that there is a bedpan in the commode before allowing the client to sit down and use it.

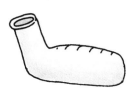

The **urinal** allows a male client to micturate without having to go to the toilet. It should be covered by a disposable cover when being transported to and from a client. Many care establishments have urinal holders that are clipped onto the side of a client's bed. They can be used by the client to hold a urinal until he is ready to use it or to store a used urinal until a member of the care staff is available to take it away. Urinals are also disposable or non-disposable, and they are disposed of and cleansed in the same way as bedpans.

Use this procedure when giving a male client a urinal:

1. Wash your hands.

2. Collect together all the necessary equipment—urinal, disposable cover, apron, and gloves.

3. Put on the plastic apron and gloves, and take the covered urinal to the client's bed.

4. Explain what you are going to do so that you can get the client's consent and cooperation.

5. Help the client into a comfortable position for using the urinal. Those who are on bedrest simply slide the urinal in place between the legs. The remainder who are allowed out of bed for short periods will stand at the side of the bed and use the urinal. The client may require help with adjusting clothing and putting the urinal in place.

6. Leave the client to use the urinal. Ensure that the call button, if required, is within easy reach.

7. Ensure privacy throughout the activity, but make sure you are in the vicinity so that you are available when the client has finished, if he requires help removing the urinal.

8. Do not try to hurry the client when he or she is using the urinal.

9. Remove the urinal, and place the cover over it.

Exercise 6.46 🖉

Managing Incontinence

Incontinence is a widespread problem. For example, it has been estimated that more than three million people in the United Kingdom suffer from incontinence to a greater or lesser degree. Faecal incontinence is less common than urinary incontinence. Incontinence is a heavy burden for the elderly. It is thought that up to one in ten adults over 65 years of age suffer occasional urinary leakage.

Incontinence, for many people, is an embarrassing subject. This is because uncontrollable leaks of urine or faeces at inconvenient times and in inconvenient places is a major cause of concern. Therefore, many people who suffer this burden will try to ignore the problem, at least initially, rather than take positive steps to try and improve the situation. Usually, the problem is only recognised when, in utter frustration and despair, a person realises that he or she can no longer hide the truth from others.

All health authorities employ one or more people who have specific responsibilities for the provision of counselling, advice, and treatment for continence problems (e.g., continence advisor, stoma therapist). Ensure that you are aware of all the resources that are available in your district to help with the maintenance of continence and/or the management of incontinence. You also need to be clear about your role in helping people with these problems.

Exercise 6.47 🖉

The main reasons an individual may choose not to seek out professional help for a continence problem include the following (Moody, 1990):

- **Fear** of not being in control and able to manage independently, fear of embarrassment or recrimination if the individual makes a mess

- **Embarrassment** at the need for help to eliminate waste products, embarrassment at having to hide the use of incontinence aids and find ways to dispose of them

- **Shame** of being incontinent and feeling dirty

- **Denial** due to fear, embarrassment, guilt, and shame, causing the individual to deny there is a problem, even in the face of overwhelming evidence (e.g., a continually wet patch on the trousers)

- **Resignation**, due to feelings of hopelessness and helplessness and the perceived inevitability of the situation

A sudden and unexpected loss of self-control resulting in incontinence is a humiliating experience that usually causes a deep sense of helplessness and shame. Many people suffer in silence, concealing the problem, even from a spouse and/or doctors. They have fears and worries about the future, and they are concerned about having the pleasures of life severely modified to cope with the problem. This can result in depression.

A person's elimination needs will start to control that individual's life. The problem dominates the person's thoughts and causes a great deal of anguish and anxiety. Any excursion from the home has to be meticulously planned to overcome the person's elimination needs, such as access to toilets, the use and disposal of incontinence pads, and the need for changes of clothing.

A positive attitude demonstrated by the care worker can go a long way to overcoming the shame, anger, hostility, or apathy shown by some clients. It is essential that the care worker avoids giving the impression of being patronising, condescending, or revolted by a client's incontinence.

The main aim of incontinence management, therefore, is to support the client in resuming a "normal" lifestyle (e.g., a lifestyle that is as near as possible to the one experienced by the person before becoming incontinent). The byword for the continence specialist is that "incontinence can sometimes be cured, usually relieved, and always made more tolerable." Support should be provided to clients in a way that promotes self-respect, maximises privacy, and is consistent with the plan of care.

Exercise 6.48

Some people are incontinent only occasionally or for a short period of time during an illness. Others are likely to have varying degrees of incontinence for the rest of their lives. The leakage of urine and/or faeces must be controlled so that it affects an individual's lifestyle as little as possible and does not damage the skin. There is a wide range of appliances, treatments, and techniques that can be considered.

Whatever method is used to manage an individual's incontinence, people are the most important resource. An individual's strengths and weaknesses will need to be identified so that a plan of care can be established to meet any self-care deficits. In a care facility, there should be few problems in providing this service. But, in the community, these needs have to be met by the family and/or other carers. This can sometimes be difficult when the family resents the incontinent person because of the restrictions on family activities imposed by the incontinence.

Incontinence Aids

A variety of incontinence aids is available. The type used by the client will depend on the continence problem and the client's capacity for self-care when using the incontinence aid.

Protective pants and pads are for intractable incontinence. They are not a cure for the problem, and an individual may regard them as such rather than seek help to overcome the root cause of the problem.

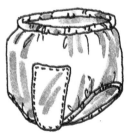

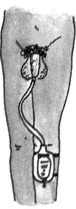

The pad that is chosen needs to be capable of absorbing the usual amount of leakage, balanced against the size of pad and type of pants that are needed to hold the pad in place, the potential for odours, and the personal preferences of the individual concerned. Other factors that need to be taken into consideration include the following:

- Client mobility and hand dexterity
- Level of alertness, mental stability to change the pad
- Vaginal/urethral discharge which may cause odours
- Type and level of faecal incontinence
- Thoroughness and regularity of hygiene measures taken by the client

Those individuals with urgency and stress incontinence, if the quantity of urine loss is small, need to have small absorbent pads that can be quickly changed. A young lady will probably want small pants that have a floral design. The older man might be quite happy with a Y front style of pants that can hold a pad. A very disabled person, with total incontinence, will require a pad capable of absorbing large amounts of urine and/or faeces.

One common mistake is thinking that several layers of pads will increase the absorbency. This will not work unless the plastic backing sheets of the pads are removed before they are put into place. Another misconception is that large pads absorb more than small pads. Less bulky pads have been developed for high absorbency.

Exercise 6.49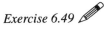

Male appliances work very well for most men, as long as they are anatomically suited to the device. Gross obesity, a retracted penis, or a scrotal hernia may make it impossible to fit a device.

A *pubic pressure urinal* is the most complicated to use as it has a number of component parts. It has a number of sizes of sheath diameters and flanges. The tip of the urinal is attached to a urine collection bag.

The *condom urinal* consists of a special sheath or condom which is attached to a urine collection bag.

Dribble bags are designed for those men who have a minor dribble incontinence. They generally consist of a disposable plastic bag on a waist band or a waterproof pouch in which to collect the urine.

All male appliances have to be washed daily by taking the appliance apart, washing well in warm, soapy water, and drying thoroughly. It is usually necessary to have several appliances so that they can be rotated.

Great care needs to be taken of the skin when wearing the appliances as they can make the penis, scrotum, and thighs sore. The appliance, when first given, should be worn for slowly increasing lengths of time until it can be well tolerated. Every time the appliance is removed, the pubic area should be thoroughly washed and dried, and inspected for any soreness. If there is any soreness, the appliance should not be re-used until full healing has occurred.

Exercise 6.50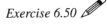

Catheters are used when all other methods of managing incontinence are considered unsuitable. The catheterisation of a client is usually only undertaken by a skilled practitioner. The catheter is kept in place by a small balloon on the catheter that is inflated inside the bladder. It is essential, therefore, that the client should not try to pull the catheter out whilst the balloon is inflated and that great care should be taken in moving these clients to ensure that tension is not placed on the catheter.

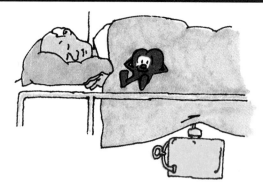

The carer needs to make sure that the catheter bag tubing is free from kinks and that it is kept below the level of the bladder so that the urine can drain freely. Usually, during the day, a client will wear a urine bag holder which can hold a catheter bag in place on the leg. At night, or when confined to bed, the catheter bag is attached to the side of the bed.

A daily bath is usually provided so that the genitals and catheter can be kept clean. The catheter bag can be detached and a spigot (bung) placed in the end of the catheter. The catheter should be carefully washed with soap and water around the urethral opening.

The catheter can be a source of urinary infection. Infected urine appears cloudy. Encourage the client to drink plenty of fluids (i.e., four pints per day). Be aware that the catheter may become blocked or the drainage can be reduced if the client is constipated. A variety of catheter bags are available that can be worn (and hidden) under the clothes.

Exercise 6.51

The most common sites for introducing an infection into a catheterised client can be seen in the diagram below.

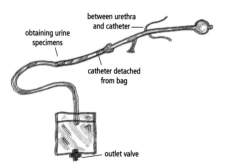

Catheter bags are emptied when necessary, rather than changed. Follow this procedure for **emptying a urinary drainage bag**:

1. Collect the necessary equipment together—swabs saturated with 70 percent isopropyl alcohol, clean jug, disposable gloves, plastic apron.

2. Wash your hands with bacteriocidal soap and water or bacteriocidal alcohol hand rub, and put on the disposable gloves and plastic apron.

3. Clean the outlet valve with a swab saturated with 70 percent isopropyl alcohol before emptying the contents of the bag into the jug.

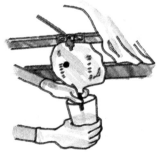

4. Close the outlet valve, and again clean it with a new swab saturated with 70 percent isopropyl alcohol.

5. Cover the jug and get rid of the contents in the sluice, having first noted the volume of urine, if this is needed for fluid balance records.

6. Wash your hands with bacteriocidal soap and water, or bacteriocidal alcohol hand rub.

Exercise 6.52

Stoma Care

A bowel or urinary stoma is usually created by a surgeon on the abdominal wall because the urinary or colonic tracts beyond the position of the stoma are damaged and no longer viable due to trauma or disease. The stoma usually appears like a slightly protruding pink/red rosebud on the abdomen. It is positioned on the abdomen so that it can be easily managed by the client. The stoma is the opening for the excretion of bowel contents or urine, depending on the operation that has been performed.

Stoma care usually focuses on the following:

- Collecting urine or bowel contents into an appropriate stoma appliance
- Maintaining good skin and stoma hygiene
- Ensuring client comfort and security with the stoma and appliances

The main cause of distress for a client who has a bowel stoma is leakage and smell. The bowel contents tend to be very malodorous. Fortunately, when appliances are fitted correctly, the client can remain odour-free. Flatus is released via charcoal filters, and deodorisers are available. Any problems that do occur, can usually be solved by the use of alternative appliances.

Exercise 6.53

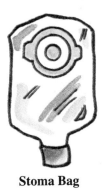

Stoma Bag

Many of the **appliances** that are now available to people who have stomas are very similar in style and effectiveness. The most essential aspect of an appliance is choosing one that is the correct size for the stoma. This is because the skin surrounding the stoma needs to be protected from the stoma output, which can be very irritable to the skin. Therefore, the appliance should fit snugly around the stoma to within 0.5 centimetres of the stoma edge. The small gap prevents the rigid appliance or its adhesive from damaging the sensitive stoma. A stoma size may change over time, requiring a change in the size of the appliance. The appliance should be leakproof and odour proof, unobtrusive (not bulky so that it is visible under clothes), noise free, and disposable.

There are two main types of appliances. The all-in-one consists of a bag with an adhesive wafer around the flange that fits around the stoma. As the bag is removed, the adhesive is separated from the skin. The two-piece appliance consists of a flange that fits around the stoma and a detachable bag. This type of device allows (potentially) sore skin to remain undisturbed.

In addition, some bags can be emptied, rather than disposed of.

The stoma is not a wound. Therefore, mild soap and water are the best cleaning agents for the stoma and surrounding skin.

Follow these guidelines for changing a stoma appliance:

1. Collect the necessary equipment— clean tray containing tissues, new appliance, and relevant accessories (e.g., filter), disposal bag, bowl of warm water and soap, jug for the contents of the old appliance, gloves, and a plastic apron.

2. Position the client to view the procedure, and place a small protective pad so that any fluid leakage does not soil the client's clothing.

3. Put on the gloves and the plastic apron.

4. If the bag is drainable, drain the contents into the jug before removing the appliance.

5. Remove the appliance by gently peeling the adhesive off the skin. Remove any mucus or faeces from the stoma area with a damp tissue.

6. Assess the stoma and surrounding skin for ulcers or soreness. Anything unusual should be reported to the person-in-charge.

7. If everything appears to be in good condition, proceed by gently washing the stoma and surrounding skin, and then gently and thoroughly drying them.

8. Apply a clean appliance. (You may remove your gloves for this task.)

9. Remove and dispose of all used equipment. In a care facility, the bag should be rinsed out with water in the sluice, wrapped in a disposable bag, and placed in an appropriate waste bin. In a client's home, the contents of the bag should be emptied down the toilet (the end of a closed bag has to be

cut off with scissors). Then the bag is flushed out with water from a jug, or by holding it under the toilet's flushing water. The bag should be wrapped in newspaper, double wrapped in plastic bags, and disposed of with the rest of the household rubbish.

10. Wash hands thoroughly, using bacteriocidal soap and water or bacteriocidal alcohol hand rub.

Exercise 6.54 ✎

Managing Sanitary Towels

From menarche to menopause, all women usually have a monthly menstrual cycle to manage. Most women cope with this natural phenomenon by wearing some kind of sanitary towel—a sanitary pad can be worn externally, or a tampon can be inserted internally. The emphasis of care for clients who are menstruating is to regularly change sanitary towels and ensure scrupulous hygiene to minimise embarrassment and odour, and to make the client as comfortable as possible.

Care should be taken with clients who have learning difficulties or who are confused. Clients have been known to forget to change their sanitary towels regularly or to insert new tampons before the soiled ones have been removed. The lack of menstrual hygiene utilised by these clients can result in genital soreness and the development of severe infections.

The majority of clients will be able to look after their own hygiene needs. When clients need help, use the following guidelines:

1. Collect the necessary equipment—clean tray containing wipes, sanitary towel disposal bag, bowl of warm water and soap, gloves, plastic apron, and protective pad.

2. Put on the gloves and plastic apron.

3. Remember that the client should be encouraged to do as much as she can for herself in relation to replacing the sanitary towel and personal hygiene.

4. Ensure privacy.

5. A small protective pad should be placed under the client so that any fluid leakage does not soil the client's bedclothes.

6. Keep the client covered as much as possible to reduce embarrassment and to keep the client warm.

7. Remove the sanitary towel. Clean the genital area with a damp wipe, and dry thoroughly.

8. Assess the genital area and the surrounding skin for soreness. Anything unusual should be reported to the person-in-charge.

9. Apply a clean sanitary towel.

10. Remove and dispose of all used equipment. The soiled sanitary towel should be placed in a sanitary towel bag for disposal in a yellow clinical waste bag, or in a sanitary towel bin or disposal unit in the toilets.

11. Wash your hands thoroughly, using bacteriocidal soap and water or bacteriocidal alcohol hand rub.

Exercise 6.55 ✎

Summary

Enabling clients to maintain their personal hygiene and appearance is an important aspect of care that promotes a feeling of well-being and helps to maintain good health. Where possible, accept other people's standards of hygiene and appearance. Whenever possible, offer clients choices that agree with their plans of care.

Where appropriate, encourage clients to switch to healthier diets. Help them to be as independent as possible in eating and drinking.

When required, accurately monitor and record clients' fluid balance. Ensure as much privacy as possible for clients to use toilet facilities. Use incontinence aids only where they are required. Take care when disposing of client waste by using Universal Precautions.

Check Your Knowledge and Understanding

1. A man has been admitted to your care facility after having a minor stroke. He cannot walk and has to be propped up in bed. He needs help with all his self-care needs. He says he would like to have a bath, but insists that the hoist is not used to get him into and out of the bath. What would you do?

   a) Insist that if the man wants to have a bath, the hoist must be used. Alternatively, he can have a bed bath.

   b) Offer the man the chance to use the shower instead.

   c) Agree to take the man to the bathroom in his wheelchair, and then slide him into and out of the bath using the wheelchair.

   d) Offer the man the chance to have a strip wash in the communal washroom.

2. You are talking to a teenage girl who says that she never has her bowels open more than once a week. What would you do?

   a) Advise the girl to start increasing the amount of roughage in her diet.

   b) Accept that the frequency of this girl's bowel actions are normal for her, unless she states that there is a problem.

   c) Ensure that a full continence assessment is carried out at the earliest opportunity.

   d) Assess the girl's dietary intake to see if that is the cause of her problem.

3. You are helping Jim, an elderly gentleman, to maintain his personal hygiene. You have helped him to brush his teeth and have a strip wash at the sink. He has three day's stubble on his chin, but claims that he does not want a shave. He also insists on putting his dirty pyjamas back on as his others are dirty and he does not like the ones provided by the home. It is obvious that Jim does not want to talk further about the subject. You know that his sister, who has previously complained about the standards of care, is visiting him that evening. What would you do?

   a) Accept that Jim has the right to refuse a shave and clean pyjamas. Then plan to intercept Jim's sister before she sees him so that you can inform her of the situation.

   b) Try your best to persuade Jim to have a shave and put on some clean pyjamas.

   c) Plan to offer Jim counselling so that you can explore why he chooses to remain unshaven and wear dirty pyjamas.

   d) Telephone Jim's sister and ask her to bring in some clean pyjamas for him, mentioning that he is choosing not to shave at the moment.

4. A client recently admitted to your care facility has recently suffered a stroke and is paralysed down her left side. She can only use her right hand to feed herself and the right side of her mouth to chew food. Although she has her food cut up for her and it is placed in a deep dish, she has problems getting the food from dish to mouth and chewing without dribbling. She is embarrassed and ashamed by this problem. How might you help?

   a) Allow the client to eat in privacy, so that none of the other clients can see her eating and drinking problems.

   b) Feed the client.

   c) Provide physical help to the client when eating and drinking. Help to get the food onto the fork or spoon, and guide the food to the client's mouth. Wipe her chin whenever she dribbles.

d) Provide the client with a non-slip table mat and plate with a clip-on, plastic plate surround to help her eat. Try offering less solid foods which can be swallowed quickly and so reduce dribbling. Wipe any dribbles from her chin immediately.

5. Michael is a middle-aged client who is recovering from a chest infection. He says that he is having trouble passing urine whilst laid in bed. Although he feels "wobbly," he would like to stand at the side of the bed to pass urine. His care plan specifies that he should rest in bed as much as possible, although he is not confined to bed. Michael has not been out of bed for the last couple of days. What would you do?

a) Allow the client to get out of bed and use the urinal in privacy.

b) Suggest that if the client wants to use the urinal at the side of the bed then there should be two care workers present and a chair behind him in case he feels faint.

c) Offer the client the use of a commode at the bedside.

d) Remind the client that, if he cannot pass urine, then he will probably need to have a urinary catheter inserted.

6. You are caring for a very overweight, elderly woman who has recently been admitted to your care facility. It soon becomes obvious that her diet consists mainly of chips, chocolate, and crisps. Unfortunately, her excessive weight is making it extremely painful for her to be mobile because of arthritis of the hip joints. The woman also has asthma, and she is often breathless. What would you do?

a) Insist that the woman commences a reducing diet "for her own good," and remove the crisps and chocolate that are stuffed in the woman's locker.

b) Accept that it is going to be very difficult to change the woman's dietary habits at her age. She has the right to eat junk food and be overweight if that is what she wants.

c) Offer the woman one of your own diet sheets so that she can start her diet straightaway.

d) Sit down with the woman and explain how her weight is aggravating her arthritis and asthma. Ask the woman if she would be willing to talk to the dietitian. Together they can plan a way to gradually reduce her intake of "junk food" and slowly replace it with healthier foods that carry less calories.

7. You are caring for a young woman who has been admitted for investigations of abdominal pain. The woman has shaved the sides of her head, and her hair is bright green. She has many facial piercings, her make-up is bright green and yellow, and she has tattoos on her forearms and hands. The rest of the clients are avoiding the woman who is sat at the side of her bed with her eyes closed listening to her personal stereo through earphones. A couple of the clients complain that "the hospital should not allow people in who look like that!" What would you do?

a) Remind the two clients who complained that the woman has the right to choose her own appearance. As long as she does not bother them, there should not be any problems.

b) Suggest to the young woman that she remove her facial piercing jewelry and cover her tattoos.

c) Transfer the woman to another clinical area where there is a side room in which she can stay.

d) Inform the woman about the complaints of the other clients so that she knows to keep well away from them.

MODULE 1

Question 1   Answer: **b**

Explanation: It should not be your decision to break the rules of confidentiality in this case. The person-in-charge will probably decide to inform the child protection officer. He or she might also want to interview the parent first and inform the parent of the intentions.

Question 2   Answer: **c**

Explanation: It is best to let the nurse-in-charge deal with this request. A patient can compel the release of computerised medical records, unless it can be contested that sight of the records could be harmful to the patient. But, most hospitals have policies to deal with this situation. Policies can include the expectation that at least two days' notice is needed before a copy of medical records is provided, and there may be a charge levied for the service.

Question 3   Answer: **d**

Explanation: You have politely tried to stop this man from harassing you. It has not worked. Therefore, it is time to take this problem further and get it sorted out.

Question 4   Answers: **a** and **b**

Explanation: The needs of the person contemplating suicide and the needs of the abused child override the need to maintain confidentiality.

Question 5   Answer: **c**

Explanation: This is the only logical alternative that will meet this man's needs to fast and your need to ensure that he consumes a good diet in order to regain some of the weight that he has lost.

Question 6   Answer: **b**

Explanation: A reprimand is likely to escalate, rather than de-escalate, the situation.

Question 7   Answer: **a**

Explanation: A clear, concise, and accurate objective report should be immediately written while the incident is still fresh in the memory.

Question 8   Answer: **c**

Explanation: If the person is only at slight risk from abuse, it is a waste of staff time to maintain constant supervision (especially if the person could be at risk for the rest of his life).

MODULE 2

Question 1   Answers: **all**

Explanation: They are all communication problems.

Question 2   Answer: **d**

Explanation: The only thing that matters is that when the lady is discharged, she takes her medication as prescribed and attends the day centre. Answer "d" is most likely to get that result.

Question 3   Answer: **b** and **c**

Explanation: Answer "b" is incorrect because nobody should be forced to use any language they do not feel comfortable using. Answer "c" is wrong because pressure should not be put on a person to talk about his problems when he is not yet ready to talk about them.

Question 4   Answer: **d**

Explanation: Reprimanding residents "a" is not the best way to form a therapeutic relationship. Ignoring the behaviour "b" is simply avoiding the problem. Moving him to a side ward and reminding carers not to bend down near him "c" is a way of managing the problem, but does not work on the source of the problem. In "d," this approach allows you to prevent the problem from happening whilst forming a positive relationship with this person and preventing him from having to be "isolated."

Question 5   Answer: **c**

Explanation: Answer "c" is an accurate, objective report. Answers "a" and "b" make assumptions that Jane is injuring herself again when there is no proof. Answer "d" is not a full report of what you know.

Question 6   Answer: **d**

Explanation: You are obviously not allowed access to this report, so you should not try to access it by other means.

Question 7   Answer: **b**

Explanation: The message is urgent. You should pass the message on to your colleague as quickly and gently as possible.

Question 8   Answer: **a**

Explanation: The message is not urgent, although it is important that the nurse receives the message that day to ensure that the patient gets another supply of tablets that day. The nurse will routinely check her desk for messages on her return, so there is no danger that she will not receive the message.

Question 9   Answer: **c**

Explanation: It makes sense not to allow anybody access to the home, never mind the residents and records, until there is proof of identification. Simply sending the social worker away would appear to be unfriendly when you can call the social work department for proof of identity.

MODULE 3

Question 1   Answer: **c**

Explanation: It is unnecessary for him to stop training "a" and "b" if he wants to maintain his fitness levels. He may be able to join in with some of the rugby training "d." Before he does so, he should get some advice on the types of training that he can undertake and how best he can support and protect his injured arm "c."

Question 2   Answer: **d**

Explanation: The emphasis in this situation is to ensure that the client can continue train spotting and overcome any "problems," if they exist, whilst ensuring that the client's rights are not infringed. Options "a" and "c" will not discover if the client's behaviour is causing a problem at the train station. Option "b" excludes the client from the assessment and planning process. Option "d" provides you with the necessary information so that an accurate assessment of the situation can be carried out and on which an action plan can be negotiated, if necessary.

Question 3   Answer: **a**

Explanation: Although the appearance of the client's brother and his two friends may appear to be a little "rough," there is no evidence that the client is likely to be abused or placed in danger during his outing. Therefore, your only option is to let the client go to the football match, as planned, although you may want to evaluate the success of the outing with the client when he returns.

Question 4   Answer: **a**

Explanation: The client's effort in writing the letter makes it obvious that he wants his own letter to be sent to his sister. Therefore, you should not demean his efforts by suggesting that you rewrite the letter "b." He has a right to have his own letter sent to his sister; therefore, you should not secretly rewrite his letter "d." It is also obvious that the client has literacy problems; therefore, it is wholly appropriate for you to address the letter and post it for him "a," rather than make the client do this for himself "c." This ensures that the letter reaches his sister.

Question 5   Answer: **c**

Explanation: There is no proof that the couple have sexually abused the child. Therefore, if you inform them of your suspicions of child abuse, before denying them permission to take the child home "a," you might unnecessarily make the couple very angry and/or upset. As a care worker, when you take the children out, you are expected to act "in loco parentis." That is, you have a legal obligation to care for the child on behalf of your employing authority. Therefore, you should not ignore the care plan and take a chance in letting the couple take the child home for an unsupervised visit "d."

Question 6   Answer: **d**

Explanation: If you inform the relatives that the client has requested that his diagnosis and treatment remain confidential, they will want to know why. If the client is ill, he will not want to be bothered by his relatives asking difficult questions about his health "b." You will breach confidentiality if you let the relatives know the client's diagnosis and treatment "c," against his wishes. This is a situation that should be managed by a care worker who has the experience and authority to sensitively handle the situation. Therefore, refer the relatives to the person- in-charge "d."

Question 7   Answer: **b**

Explanation: If the home has an appropriate philosophy of care, it should not have a very strict routine, and it should not try to exclude family and friends from providing care for residents. Therefore, you should not comply with the care staff's wishes "a." You could make a formal complaint "c," but this is likely to create a bad atmosphere and may not improve the situation. You may feel like withdrawing your relative from the home "d," but this might be premature if your relative is receiving good quality care and if the care staff are willing to show flexibility in involving you in the provision of care "b."

Question 8   Answer: **c**

Explanation: The couple may or may not claim welfare benefits in the future "a," but if they are likely to suffer due to inadequate finances, you should inform your supervisor and see if they are willing to talk through their financial problems with an appropriately qualified officer "c." Unless you have the appropriate experience and training, it would not be appropriate for you to review the couple's finances "b." You do not have the right to insist that the carer does anything, even when your motives are positive "d."

MODULE 4

Question 1   Answer: **c**

Explanation: You need to conduct a thorough search "c," before implementing the missing person procedure "a" or contacting the police "d." If you wait to see if he wanders back on his own "b," he could hurt himself badly.

Question 2   Answer: **c**

Explanation: Answer "c" is the only safe alternative. Just because you cannot see flames or smoke does not mean that there is not a fire. The fire brigade would rather be called out to a fire at this stage than to a blazing inferno. They will not be angry if it is a false alarm.

Question 3   Answer: **d**

Explanation: A carer who has not yet completed the lifting and moving course "d" should not be involved in the lifting and moving of clients. The drag lift "a" should never be used because it is likely to result in harm to the carers and/or the client. You are not qualified to teach the new carer how to move a client up the bed "b," and you should never try to lift a person up in bed by yourself "c."

Question 4   Answer: **c**

Explanation: Answer "c" is the most appropriate answer. Answer "b" is second best because it may be quite a while before these people can be released for the AIDS workshop. Answer "a" is simply an unhelpful comment. Answer "d" is incorrect.

Question 5   Answer: **c**

Explanation: Answer "c" is the correct, immediate, first-aid treatment for a burn.

Question 6   Answer: **a**

Explanation: If the person is hypoglycaemic as you suspect, the sweets will allow him to recover quickly. If the person does not recover quickly, call the doctor. All other options are highly dangerous.

MODULE 5

Question 1   Answer: **b**

Explanation: Pain is what the client says it is. Therefore, it would not be appropriate to ask the client if he has a low pain/discomfort threshold "a" or point out to the client that he is the only one of the six clients who have undergone the same investigative procedure that is complaining of pain "d." Once you have informed the person-in-charge, she will ensure that the pain is appropriately assessed "b." In a hospital, pain assessment is usually undertaken by the nurses, rather than the health care support workers. The doctor can then be informed of the situation. You cannot ask the person-in-charge to provide you with some analgesia for the client "c" as he has not been prescribed any analgesia or been assessed by either the nurse or the doctor.

Question 2   Answer: **a**

Explanation: The client may be happy simply sticking with her current medication "b" or seeking a smaller sized analgesic tablet "d." It would be inappropriate to suggest that she only takes the analgesic tablets when her face is very painful "c" as that would leave her with untreated mild pain which is very fatiguing and which might make her life miserable. The best suggestion, though, is for the client to try an alternative method of pain relief "a" for the mild pain which reduces her taking of tablets to a minimum.

Question 3   Answers: **d**

Explanation: Answer "d" is the only option. Answer "a" is inappropriate because all lifting is to be avoided where possible. Answer "c" risks hurting both the client and you. Answer "b" cannot be right if the member of care staff is refusing to use the available slide sheets. You should inform your manager about the member of staff who is wanting to lift clients and who is refusing to use the available manual handling aids.

Question 4   Answer: **a**

Explanation: The only option that is a safe manual handling strategy, both for the client and the care staff, is "a." Don't forget to inform the person-in-charge of this problem and your chosen solution in case the client decides to complain.

Question 5   Answer: **c**

Explanation: Whilst it would not be appropriate to insist that this client continues her active and passive exercises "a" and "b" when she is expected to die in the next couple of days, you simply cannot leave her alone to deteriorate "d" as this is likely to make her last days of life very uncomfortable. Therefore, you should sit down with the client (and family, if appropriate) to discuss a plan of care which ensures that she remains as comfortable as possible until she dies.

Question 6   Answer: **c**

Explanation: There is still some movement left in the client's left arm and leg, so the situation is not hopeless "d," although you would want the client to do as much as he can for himself. It would not be appropriate to implement an active exercise regime for the client "b" until he has been properly assessed by the physiotherapist "a." Unfortunately, because it may be a while before the physiotherapist can come to assess the client, you will need to implement some action in the meantime to prevent the client's left arm and leg from deteriorating further "c."

Question 7   Answer: **c**

Explanation: Until a full assessment has been carried out, you cannot be sure what the problem is or how it should be treated/managed. A full assessment needs to be carried out before you can devise a plan of care for this problem.

MODULE 6

Question 1   Answer: **a**

Explanation: The only option that is a safe manual handling strategy, both for the client and the care staff, is "a." Don't forget to inform the person-in-charge of this problem and your chosen solution in case the client decides to complain.

Question 2   Answer: **b**

Explanation: There is a wide range of normal frequency of bowel actions. For this girl, one bowel action per week is normal and it does not seem to be causing her any problems. Therefore, no assessment or intervention appears to be necessary.

Question 3   Answer: **d**

Explanation: Jim has the right to refuse a shave and clean pyjamas. Whilst it would be appropriate to try and intercept Jim's sister "a" before she sees him so that you can inform her of the situation, the best approach is to telephone Jim's sister "d" and ask her to bring in some clean pyjamas for him, mentioning that he is choosing not to shave at the moment. This acknowledges Jim's rights to self-determination and overcomes the problem of him not having any clean pyjamas. You should not offer Jim counselling "c" when he is obviously not in the mood to talk.

Question 4   Answer: **d**

Explanation: Although eating in privacy "a" may seem to be a good solution to the client's embarrassment, meal times are normally social occasions and if the source of the client's embarrassment can be removed or reduced, she may be happy to eat and drink in the company of others. Feeding the client "b" and providing physical assistance to eat and drink "c" are not appropriate as they do not encourage independence when the client can feed herself.

Question 5   Answer: **b**

Explanation: The catheter "d" is the last option in helping most clients meet their elimination needs. The client should be allowed to use the urinal whilst stood at the side of the bed, but not in privacy "a" for the moment, as he has been in bed for two days, says he feels "wobbly" and, therefore could feel feint whilst using the urinal. If there are two care workers stood at his side and a chair behind him "b," this is the safe way for the client to use the urinal whilst stood at the side of the bed. If the client does feel somewhat feint whilst using the urinal, it may then be appropriate to try a commode "c."

Question 6   Answer: **d**

Explanation: You cannot insist that the woman commences a diet "a," even if it is "for her own good." You should not offer the woman one of your own diet sheets "c" when there is a dietitian available who can provide the woman with a diet sheet to more specifically meet her needs. Although it may be very difficult to change this woman's dietary habits "b," an effort should be made to try to persuade the woman to eat a healthier diet. The dietitian "d" is the specialist who should do this.

Question 7   Answer: **a**

Explanation: The woman has the right to choose her own appearance "a," however inappropriate the care staff or the other clients may think it is. You should not show prejudice by suggesting that she removes her jewelry "b," or by transferring the woman to a side room in another clinical area "c," or by expecting the woman to keep well away from the clients who have complained about her appearance "d."

Suggested Reading

Bornat J et al (eds) (1998) **Community Care: A Reader**. MacMillan: Basingstoke.

Burnard P (1992) **Effective Communication Skills for the Health Professions**. Chapman & Hall: London.

Department for Education and Employment (1995) **Disability Discrimination Act**. HMSO: London.

Department of Health (1992) **Health of the Nation**. HMSO: London.

Department of Health (1995) **On the State of the Public Health** 1994. HMSO: London.

Department of Health (1995) **The Patient's Charter and You**. HMSO: London.

Douglas A et al (1998) **Service Users' Perspectives on "Floating" Support**. Joseph Rowntree Foundation: York.

Equal Opportunities Commission (1986) **Guidelines for Equal Opportunities Employers**. EOC: London.

Getliffe K & Dolman M (eds) (1997) **Promoting Continence: A Clinical and Research Resource**. Balliere Tindall: London.

Griffiths-Jones A & Ward K (1995) **Principles of Infection Control Practice**. Scutari Press: London.

Karmi G (1998) **Ethnicity, Health and Society**. Blackwell Science: Oxford.

Mallett J & Bailey C (eds) (1996) **The Royal Marsden NHS Trust Manual of Clinical Nursing Procedures** (4th ed). Blackwell Science: Oxford.

Moody M (1990) **Incontinence: Patient Problems and Nursing Care**. Heinemann Nursing: Oxford.

Myerscough P R & Ford M (1996) **Talking With Patients: Keys to Good Communication**. Oxford medical Publication: Oxford.

National Health Service Estates (1995) **Health Guidance Note: Safe Disposal of Clinical Waste Whole Hospital Policy Guidance**. HMSO: London.

Resuscitation Council (1997) **The 1997 Resuscitation Huidelines for Use in the United Kingdom**. Resuscitation Council: London.

Royal College of Nursing (1997) **The Handling of Patients** (4th ed). RCN: London.

Royal College of Nursing & National Back Pain Association (1998) **The Guide to the Handling of Patients**. RCN: London.

St John's Ambulance, St Andrew's Ambulance Association & British Red Cross (1995) **First Aid**. Dorling Kindersley: London.

Tadd V (1998) **Ethics and Values for Carers**. Blackwell Science: Oxford.

Thompson N (1997) **Anti-Discriminatory Practice** (2nd ed). MacMillan: Basingstoke.

United Kingdom Central Council for Nursing, Midwifery and Health Visiting (1987) **Confidentiality: An Elaboration of Clause 9**. UKCC: London.

United Kingdom Central Council for Nursing, Midwifery and Health Visiting (1992) **Standards for the Administration of Medicines**. UKCC: London.

Wilkinson R G (1996) **Unhealthy Societies: The Affliction of Inequality**. Routledge: London.

Wilson J (1995) **Infection Control in Clinical Practice**. Harcourt Brace & Co: London.

Wright F (1998) **The Effect on Carers of a Frail Older Person's Admission to a Care Home**. Joseph Rowntree Foundation: York.

References

Department of Employment (1974) **Health and Safety at Work Act**. HMSO: London.

Department of the Environment (1990) **Environmental Protection Act**. HMSO: London.

Department of Health (1990) **The NHS and Community Care Act**. HMSO: London.

Department of Health (1997) **The New NHS: Modern, Dependable**. HMSO: London.

Department of Trade and Industry (1994) **The Control of Substances Hazardous to Health Regulations**. HMSO: London.

Health and Safety Commission (1987) **Violence to Staff in the Health Services**. HMSO: London.

Home Office (1998) **The Data Protection Act** 1998. HMSO: London.

Poyner B & Warne C (1988) **Health and Safety Executive Report: Preventing Violence to Staff**. HMSO: London.

Robinson J R & Elkan R (1996) **Health Needs Assessment: Theory and Practice**. Churchill Livingstone: New York.

United Nations (1948) **Universal Declaration of Human Rights**. UN: Geneva.

United Nations (1971) **Declaration on the Rights of Mentally Retarded Persons**. UN: Geneva.

Wondrak R (1989) **Dealing with Verbal Abuse**. Nurse EducationToday, 9, 276-280.

Glossary

A

abuse mental, physical, sexual, medical, or financial abuse, exploitation, or neglect

acidosis disturbance of normal metabolism that causes body fluids to become more acidic than normal

acupuncture procedure whereby needles are inserted into specific points on a body in order to achieve a desired effect

adopted role set of behaviours and responsibilities taken on by a person who accepts a specified role (e.g., new job)

advocate someone who speaks up on behalf of, and the benefit of, another person

alimentary canal body canal into which food and drink is inserted at the top end (mouth), and faeces is excreted at the bottom end; digestion takes place along the way

analgesic medication that reduces the level of pain

angina severe, but temporary attack of cardiac pain, usually caused by exercise in people with heart disease

antibody specific substances produced in the blood, in response to being in contact with foreign protein, that have a role in the development of immunity

anus the end of the alimentary canal at the termination of the rectum; consists of a sphincter muscle which allows the excretion of faeces

anxiety attack sudden bout of feelings of fear, apprehension, and dread, often referred to as panic attacks

aphasia difficulty using or understanding words

articulation ability to speak clearly

ascribed role set of behaviours and responsibilities that are assigned to a person because of his or her association with a specific group (e.g., an individual born into the royal household)

aseptic technique no-touch technique using sterile instruments during invasive clinical procedures that prevents susceptible body sites from becoming contaminated by pathogenic bacteria

assault unlawful personal attack

assertiveness refers to a confident and direct (but non-threatening and polite) way of powerfully communicating with others in a positive fashion, without denying their rights

at risk exposed to hazard or danger

audit formal inspection and assessment for the purposes of reporting and making recommendations for change

autoclave machine that uses high pressure steam to achieve sterilisation

B

BP blood pressure

bacteriocidal describes any agent that destroys bacteria

battery attack where an actual blow is delivered

C

CPR cardiopulmonary resuscitation

catheter hollow tube of variable length and bore that is used for the introduction or withdrawal of fluid from body cavities

cellulose carbohydrate from the outer walls of plant and vegetable cells; cannot be digested by man and, therefore, provides roughage

challenging behaviour problem behaviour that is demanding and disruptive, which makes it difficult to provide quality support and care

claustrophobia form of mental disturbance where there is a morbid fear of confined spaces

colitis inflammation of the colon

colon large bowel

colostomy	surgically created opening between the colon (large bowel) and the surface of the abdomen
communication	act of conveying information to another person via speech, signs, symbols, touch, or writing
complementary health services	examples include massage, osteopathy, acupuncture, aroma therapy, and reflexology
confidentiality	non-disclosure of information in order to maintain the privacy/secrecy of spoken, written, or electronic facts
confusion	used to describe the mental state of a person who is out of touch with reality; may be associated with a clouding of consciousness
crepitus	sound when two broken ends of a bone scrape together
crisis	point in time when an urgent and stressful situation is overwhelming to a person
Crohn's disease	chronic inflammatory disease of the bowel
cross-infection	becoming infected by a new or different micro-organism transferred from equipment or another person
cystitis	inflammation of the internal wall of the resulting in frequency and urgency in passing urine

D

data	accumulated information or facts
deep venous thrombosis	refers to the formation of a blood clot in one of the leg veins, usually due to poor circulation and lack of movement; can result in a pulmonary embolism
defamation	falsehoods (libel or slander) that result in damage to a person's reputation or character
defibrillation	a controlled electric shock from a machine, applied over the heart, to try and restart it or to stop it from beating abnormally
dementia	serious mental deterioration

dental caries	tooth decay
depersonalisation	effect on a person of an institutionalised environment in which there is little opportunity for individual expression (e.g., lack of personal possessions, no privacy)
discrimination	perceived differences (usually showing a preference) between alternatives
disinfection	destruction of the majority of micro-organisms on inanimate objects by the use of disinfectant
disorientation	mild state of confusion where a person becomes lost or unfamiliar with the familiar
diuretic	substance which stimulates the body to produce more urine
diversionary activity	activity which is undertaken to focus the mind away from something unpleasant or to stop a person from becoming bored
diversity	different or varied
drug dependence	situation where an individual becomes psychologically or physically reliant on a drug being administered in order to prevent the appearance of withdrawal symptoms
drug tolerance	situation where increasing amounts of a drug have to be given to achieve the same effect

E

e-mail	electronic mail: a method of sending an electronic copy of a letter and/or documents between computers that have been networked (connected together)
eczema	non-contagious skin condition which is often described as a reaction to an irritant by an already susceptible skin
empathy	ability to communicate to another person that you understand his or her feelings whilst demonstrating acceptance, respect, and trust
encopresis	incontinence of faeces
enema	injection of fluid into the rectum
enuresis	incontinence of urine, usually applied to bed wetting

epilepsy	disorder of the brain where abnormal electrical discharges cause disruption to brain functions and can result in a "fit"
equality	having identical privileges, rights, or status
excretion	elimination of waste material from the body
expectoration	act of coughing up and spitting out lung secretions (sputum)
exudate	oozing out of fluid from small blood vessels or sweat from the pores of the skin

F

false documentation	entries in a personal record that are not true
fax	method of sending a document on a telephone line between fax machines so that an (almost) exact copy of the document that was sent can be reproduced by the recipient fax machine
first aid	emergency care, before medical help arrives, for a person who is ill or injured
flatus	bowel gas, abdominal/colonic wind
fluid balance	the idea that the human body has to intake enough fluids to at least match those that are being lost from the body in urine, faeces, respiration, sweat, etc.

G

granulation tissue	outgrowth of new blood vessels and connective tissue cells from the surface of an open wound that is healing

H

haemorrhoids	dilated blood vessels that grow inside the rectum, making defaecation painful
halo effect	tendency to conform to others' expectations
Heimlich manoeuvre	first aid procedure for airway obstruction
hives	allergic skin reaction that looks like nettle rash
homeopathy	method of treating disease by prescribing minute doses of naturally occurring substances

hyper-glycaemia	higher than normal level of glucose in the blood
hypo-allergenic	very unlikely to cause an allergic reaction
hypo-glycaemia	lower than normal level of glucose in the blood

I

ileostomy	surgically created opening between the ileum (small bowel) and the surface of the abdomen
institutional-isation	effect on a person who lives in an environment where there is rigidity of routine, block treatment, depersonalisation, and little opportunity to express individuality
Internet	world-wide network of databases and connections through which information can be accessed and passed to others via computers
interpersonal skills	ability to communicate and develop a rapport with other people
invasive	describes clinical activities that bypass the body's natural defences to infection

K

ketones	substances produced by incomplete metabolism, which can cause acidosis

L

label	classifying word or phrase that identifies something
lesion	pathological change in body tissue
lethargy	state of listlessness and lack of energy
libel	written, defamatory statement

M

menarche	point in a girl's life when she starts to menstruate and becomes fertile
menopause	point in a woman's life when menstruation no longer occurs and she is no longer fertile
mental defence mechanism	mental distortion of fact to protect oneself from stressful thoughts and feelings

microbiology	science relating to micro-organisms
micro-organisms	living organisms that can only be seen with a microscope (e.g., bacteria, viruses, some fungi)
micturition	act of passing urine
modulation	adjustments and regulation of the tone of voice during conversation

N

negligence	failure to give assigned care, or giving improper care that causes harm (e.g., failure to raise bed rails, resulting in someone falling out of bed)
netelast	very flexible, tubular gauze that is used for holding dressings in place
nocturia	need to pass urine that wakes a person during the night
non-compliance	refusal to do what one has been asked to do
non-sedentary	describes activities that involve physical effort
non-verbal communication	non-spoken information that is purposely or accidentally conveyed to another person during an interaction (e.g., facial expression, gestures, posture)
norm	usual for a given situation

O

oedema	abnormal swelling of tissues due to retention of fluid
oesophagus	canal through which food is swallowed, extending from the back of the throat down to the stomach
orthosis	piece of equipment which is worn to help provide support to parts of the body (e.g., surgical shoes)

P

paranoia	delusions (false perceptions) of persecution
pathology	science related to the cause and nature of disease

peak flow	greatest amount of air that can be expelled from the lungs after taking the deepest breath possible
perianal	area around the anus
podiatry	care of the feet (chiropody)
prejudice	unfavourable opinion formed without proper judgment
prognosis	forecast about the course or outcome of an illness
prostate gland	male gland through which the urethra passes on leaving the bladder
prosthesis	piece of equipment that replaces a missing body part (e.g., artificial limb)
protective barriers	coverings to guard against infection (e.g., gloves, masks, aprons)
psoriasis	chronic, non-contagious, skin disease where inflamed areas of skin are covered in silvery scales
pulmonary embolism	blood clot that travels to the blood vessels of the lung (potentially fatal)

Q

quadriplegia	paralysis of all four limbs

R

radiography	process of imaging (e.g., X-rays)
rapport	harmonious accord; relationship that makes communication possible or easy
reflection	relates to a conscious process of thinking and interpreting experience in order to learn from it
relaxation therapy	to make or become less tense, where there is stimulation of that part of the nervous system that results in relaxation
rights	legal and/or moral entitlements; what is due to a person
roughage	that part of food and drink intake that contains cellulose, providing bulk in the diet which stimulates peristalsis and the elimination of waste products

sacral area	skin and tissue above the sacrum at the base of the spine, on which you sit	stigma	unpleasant or disgraceful characteristics attached to a person or group of people
sebaceous glands	small glands in the skin that secrete oil into hair follicles and onto the body surface	stoma	surgical opening connecting a body passage with the outside (e.g., colostomy, urostomy)
sedentary	describes activities that involve no (or very little) physical effort	stress	mental, emotional, or physical strain or tension
senile dementia	irreversible deterioration in a person's mental faculties due to old age	stroke	rupture of a blood vessel in the brain; often results in paralysis and damage to speech

T

seizure	abnormal functioning of the brain, often including loss of consciousness, caused by abnormal electrical discharges within the brain	TENS	transcutaneous electric nerve stimulation
		TPR	temperature, pulse, and respiration
sharps	needles and other sharp objects (e.g., glass)	therapeutic relationship	enabling relationship in which a carer helps another person to meet his or her own needs
side effect	any unwanted effect of a treatment after administration of a drug, that does not necessarily restrict its use	toxicity	dangerous effects of a drug treatment that are usually dose related
significant other	relative, friend, or anyone who is important to another person	tumour	swelling caused by a mass of abnormal tissue which resembles normal tissue, but fulfills no useful function and can be harmful
skin flora	micro-organisms that have adapted to live on the skin of a host		

U

slander	spoken, defamatory statement	unconditional positive regard	relationship in which warmth, acceptance, and empathy are freely given
sphincter	circular muscle which can be contracted or relaxed to close or open a body orifice (e.g.,anus)	Universal Precautions	safety measures used with blood and body fluids
spirometry	the measurement of lung volumes of gas	ureter	duct that provides a passage for urine from the kidney to the bladder
sporicidal	lethal to the spores (seeds) of bacteria	urethra	passage leading from the bladder to the outside world through which urine is passed
sputum	the secretions that are coughed up from the lungs	urostomy	surgically created opening onto the surface of the abdomen through which urine can be voided
stereotype	characteristics which are held to be common to members of a category		

V

sterile	free from all micro-organisms	verbal communication	refers to spoken communication (e.g., words, language, tone of voice)
sterilisation	process of killing all living micro-organisms, usually by heat treatment		

Level 2 NVQ/SVQ Requirements

Mandatory Group A Units

- Contribute to the protection of individuals from abuse.

- Promote effective communication and relationships.

- Promote people's equality, diversity, and rights.

- Promote, monitor, and maintain health, safety, and security in the workplace.

Option Group B Units

- Contribute to the movement and handling of individuals to maximise their physical comfort.

- Contribute to the ongoing support of clients and others significant to them.

- Enable clients to access and use toilet facilities.

- Enable clients to achieve physical comfort.

- Enable clients to maintain and improve their mobility through exercise and the use of mobility appliances.

- Enable clients to maintain their personal hygiene and appearance.

- Promote communication with individuals where there are communication differences.

- Enable clients to eat and drink.

- Promote communication with individuals where there are communication differences.

- Receive, transmit, store, and retrieve information.

- Support individuals experiencing changes in their care requirements and provision.

Please note that most of the level 2 NVQ/SVQ units included within this workbook are also components of the old level 2 NVQ/SVQ in Care awards and some of them are also component units of other level 2 and 3 NVQ/SVQ awards:

- Blood Donor Support (level 2)

- Care (level 3)

- Caring for Children and Young People (level 3)

- Diagnostic and Therapeutic Support (level 3)

- Dialysis Support (level 3)

- Operating Department Support (level 2)

- Health Care - Technical Cardiology (level 2)

- Health Care - Technical Cardiology (level 3)

- Health Care Physiological Measurement - Audiology (level 3)

- Health Care Physiological Measurement - Neurophysiology (level 3)

- Health Care Physiological Measurement - Respiratory (level 3)

- Promoting Independence (level 3)

All care support workers who actively provide care services for other people should have the chance to achieve accreditation for the work that they do. It is expected that legislation will soon be proposed that expects all care workers to have achieved, or to be working towards achieving, an appropriate SVQ/NVQ in Care.

The level 2 NVQ/SVQ in Care Award is appropriate for a wide variety of care support workers:

- Newly employed and inexperienced care support workers who have not yet mastered the care roles expected of them

- Experienced care support workers who wish to have their competence formally accredited

Please Note:

It is essential to remember that you, as a care support worker, are under the indirect or direct supervision of a qualified care professional. A professionally qualified care practitioner must retain accountability for the assessment planning and review of care, for ensuring standards of care, and for determining the activity of support staff. It is important that you should not be expected or allowed to work beyond your level of competence.

Index